The NutriBase Guide to

FAST-FOOD
NUTRITION

D1554836

The NutriBase Guide to

FAST-FOOD
NUTRITION

AVERY
a member of Penguin Putnam Inc.
NEW YORK

Most Avery books are available at special quantity discounts for bulk purchase for sales promotions, premiums, fund-raising, and educational needs. Special books or book excerpts also can be created to fit specific needs. For details, write Putnam Special Markets, 375 Hudson Street, New York, NY 10014.

a member of
Penguin Putnam Inc.
375 Hudson Street
New York, NY 10014
www.penguinputnam.com

Library of Congress Cataloging-in-Publication Data

The NutriBase guide to fast-food nutrition—2nd ed.
p. cm.
ISBN 1-58333-108-5
1. Convenience foods—Composition—Tables. 2. Food—Composition—Tables.
TX551 .N745 2001   2001046274
613.2'8—dc21

Printed in the United States of America
7 9 10 8

CONTENTS

INTRODUCTION

For thousands of years, people have recognized the life-sustaining nature of food. But only during the last four or five decades have we begun to understand the many ways in which our choices of foods can affect the quality of our health and the length of our lives. And only during the last five or ten years have we really begun to appreciate how profound the effects of those choices can be.

Now we know that some of the so-called "inevitable" diseases, such as atherosclerosis, osteoporosis, and even cancer are often the consequence of poor nutritional choices. Research has clearly shown the relationship between poor nutritional intake and many of these diseases. The studies prove that a high-fat diet can—and often does—contribute to the development of coronary artery disease; that low fiber intake promotes the development of colon cancer; that folic acid deficiency increases the risk of birth defects; and that inadequate calcium intake fosters the onset of osteoporosis and bone fractures. The list of nutrition-related disorders goes on and on.

There is a hopeful side to this story. Studies have clearly demonstrated the positive effects that good nutritional choices can have on our health. Many cases of cardiovascular disease can be prevented, and even reversed, through dietary changes. The incidence of cancer can be reduced with diets that are low in fat and high in cruciferous vegetables (broccoli and cauliflower, for instance) and through the use of the antioxidant nutrients, such as vitamins C and E. Bone strength can be increased and fracture rates decreased with a diet rich in calcium and vitamin D. Blood cholesterol levels can be reduced with dietary fiber, niacin, and garlic. Blood pressure can be lowered with sodium restriction and calcium and magnesium supplementation. The list of health-promoting nutritional interventions is lengthy and is growing constantly.

THE NEW NUTRITION

Modern research studies are giving rise to a "new" nutrition, one that is both scientifically sound and practical. The new nutrition differs from the old in at least two important ways. First, the old nutrition dealt in generalities, such as the four food groups, and created minimum dietary recommendations designed to prevent deficiency-related disorders. The new nutrition seeks to achieve *optimal* levels of health and creates specific recommendations based on individual differences, such as age, sex, lifestyle, and medical factors. Second, the old nutrition left many nutritional decisions up to the health professionals and food marketers, while new nutrition puts *you* in control. It empowers you with the information necessary to evaluate confusing and conflicting claims, and it enables you to reject foods that do not meet your nutritional needs and goals.

This book is designed to provide you with that empowering information. It will help you make wiser choices when you buy food and when you dine out. It will help you interpret nutritional stories in the media so you can distinguish useful information from nonsense. It will give you the control you need over your personal nutrition.

Many people refer to books of this sort as "counter" books, because of the nutritional numbers that fill the pages. But this is not a book about counting. This is a book about *control* and *choices*. Use this book to learn more about the foods you should consume—or avoid—so you can meet your particular nutritional needs. Don't be intimidated by the huge number of choices listed or by all the nutritional value numbers that accompany the lists. It is not necessary to memorize these numbers.

Instead, just try to familiarize yourself with the foods and food categories that are best suited to your needs. Begin by looking up the foods that you eat most often or in the largest quantities. If these foods are not providing you with the nutrients you need, use the book to find better alternatives that are just as tasty. Once you are familiar with the nutritional content of your most common food choices, gradually look up the remainder of the foods in your diet. You'll be surprised by how easy it is to learn about these foods and to make any necessary changes.

As you take more control over the foods you are eating and put more thought into your choices, keep in mind that good nutrition is just one element of a healthy lifestyle. To achieve maximum benefits from the new nutrition, your life should be filled with physical activity and free of cigarette smoke and other toxic substances. In addition, the stress in your life should be under control. Even the best diet can't overcome the problems caused by smoking, an immoderate use of alcohol, poorly managed stress, or other health-compromising habits.

Finally, be aware that research is constantly adding to our knowledge of nutrition and in the process changing some of our beliefs. As best you can, try to keep up with the new information and, when appropriate, make whatever dietary changes are necessary. But also be skeptical about nutritional news that seems too good to be true. (More often than not, it isn't true.) Be wary of nutritional claims made by people who are trying to sell you something. And be cautious—don't make any drastic changes in your nutritional program without first talking to a health professional who is knowledgeable about nutrition and about your particular medical circumstances. Don't forget: If the right nutritional choices are powerful enough to keep you well, it is only logical that the wrong ones could make you sick.

The following section will explain some of the basics of nutrition. After that, you will learn how to use this book to locate the information you need to improve your diet.

A QUICK LOOK AT THE BASIC NUTRIENTS AND MICRONUTRIENTS

Everyone's diet must contain the four basic nutrients—water, complex carbohydrates, protein, and fats—as well as the micronutrients, which are the vitamins and minerals. These nutrients and micronutrients fuel the body and enable all bodily functions to occur. A proper balance of these essentials is necessary for optimum health.

This book presents the nutrient values of a wide range of foods, both whole and processed. In order to wisely use this information, it is important to have a basic understanding of the function of the nutrients and micronutrients needed by the body.

The Nutrients

Water, complex carbohydrates, protein, and fats are the basic building blocks of a healthy diet. Each works in different ways to fuel the body, build and repair the cells that make up the body, and provide the environment in which the cells live.

Water

The human body is two-thirds water by weight. Indeed, water is an essential nutrient that is involved in every function of the body. It helps transport nutrients and waste products into and out of cells. It is necessary for all digestive, absorptive, circulatory, and excretory functions, and for the utilization of the water-soluble vitamins. And it is needed to maintain proper body temperature.

Most of us are aware of some of the early signs of dehydration: scant or dark urine, thirst, and a dry mouth. If the body continues to be denied adequate water, serious health problems can occur, necessitating hospitalization.

Complex Carbohydrates

Complex carbohydrates provide the body with the energy it needs to function. Signs of an inadequate supply of complex carbohydrates include lack of energy and the breakdown of proteins in tissues.

One type of carbohydrate you may have heard a good deal about is fiber. Referred to in the past as roughage, fiber is actually the part of plant material that our body cannot digest. Yet fiber is known to perform a number of important functions. It promotes feelings of fullness; prevents constipation, hemorrhoids, and other intestinal problems; and is associated with a reduced incidence of colon cancer. In addition, fiber may help lower blood cholesterol levels, reducing the risk of heart disease.

Protein

Protein is essential for growth and development. It provides the body with energy, and is needed for the manufacture of hormones, antibodies, enzymes, and muscle tissues. It also helps maintain the proper acid-alkali balance. Inadequate protein intake can result in stunted growth, diarrhea, vomiting, lack of appetite, and edema, a buildup of fluids in the tissues.

Fats

Much attention has been focused on the need to limit dietary fat intake. Nevertheless, the body does need fats—but the right fats, and in appropriate quantities. Specifically, it needs essential fatty acids, which perform a variety of vital bodily functions. Essential fatty acids carry the fat-soluble vitamins. They are essential for growth and development, and for the maintenance of healthy skin, hair, and nails. And they provide the body with energy. A variety of problems can occur if the body fails to receive adequate amounts of essential fatty acids. Signs of deficiency may include retarded growth; skin, hair, and nail disorders; and an impaired metabolism of fats and fat-soluble vitamins.

Most of us are aware that there are several kinds of dietary fat—saturated, polyunsaturated, and monounsaturated—and that some are better than others. To understand the difference between these three types of fats, it is helpful to first learn a little about cholesterol.

Cholesterol is a white, waxy, fatty substance produced by the liver. It is essential to our well-being, as it helps to build cell membranes, to produce hormones, and to manufacture bile acids. The liver is capable of manufacturing all of the cholesterol needed for good health.

The cholesterol manufactured by the liver is carried through the bloodstream by molecules known as low-density lipoproteins, or LDLs. High levels of LDLs in the bloodstream are associated with clogged arteries, high blood pressure, stroke, and heart disease. This is why LDL is sometimes referred to as "bad cholesterol." Fortunately, many people can reduce their LDL levels through proper diet.

High-density lipoproteins, or HDLs, are molecules that carry excess cholesterol from different body tissues back to the liver, where the cholesterol is converted into bile acids and then eliminated through the intestines. High levels of HDLs are linked with a decreased risk of cardiovascular disease. This is why HDL is often called "good cholesterol." To a limited extent, HDL levels can be raised through regular exercise.

How are the three types of fats related to cholesterol? Saturated fats—which come from foods of animal origin such as meat, fish, poultry, milk, butter, and cheese, as well as from palm, coconut, and palm kernel oil—have been shown to increase total blood cholesterol levels, especially the undesirable LDL portion. Polyunsaturated fats—found mainly in vegetable oils like corn, sunflower, safflower, and soybean—tend to lower levels of both HDL and LDL. Monounsaturated fats—found mainly in certain vegetable and nut oils, including olive, peanut, and canola—have been shown to reduce total blood cholesterol without lowering levels of the good cholesterol, HDL. Indeed, some monounsaturated fats have been shown to raise HDL levels.

Most experts agree that it is best to limit fat consumption and to choose mostly monounsaturated fats, which increase the levels of HDL while lowering total blood cholesterol. There is, in fact, no biological need for saturated fat!

A Word About Calories

When we talk about foods, we often mention the number of calories a certain food has. Calories are not among the four basic nutrients, nor are they considered micronutrients. What, then, are calories?

A calorie is an energy unit. As already discussed, carbohydrates, protein, and fats provide the body with the energy it needs to function. This energy is measured in calories. There are, for instance, approximately four calories in every gram of protein, four calories in every gram of carbohydrate, and nine calories in every gram of fat. It is no wonder, then, that people who are trying to lose weight are often advised to cut down on fatty foods. On a gram-for-gram basis, fat is more than twice as fattening as carbohydrates or protein.

In addition to having more calories than protein or carbohydrates, dietary fat is metabolized differently. Because dietary fat is similar in chemical composition to body fat, it takes less energy to convert it to body fat. In fact, it takes only 3 percent of the calories in the fat we eat to turn that food into body fat, while it takes at least 25 percent of the calories in the carbohydrates and protein we eat to convert them into body fat. Remember, though, that if you eat more calories than your body needs, regardless of the nutrient source of these calories, the excess will be stored as body fat.

Being Sodium Wise

Not even a brief look at nutrition would be complete without a word or two about sodium. The mineral sodium is necessary for health. It helps maintain normal fluid levels in the body, is involved in healthy muscle functioning, and supports the blood and lymphatic systems.

It is important to note, however, that most people get too much sodium in their diets. We need less than 500 milligrams of sodium a day to stay healthy. This is enough to accomplish the functions that sodium performs in the body. A quick glance through some randomly selected pages of this book will show you how easy it is to reach the 500-milligram mark. You may be surprised by the amount of salt present in the foods you eat regularly and by your typical daily intake.

THE FOOD GUIDE PYRAMID

Because the four basic nutrients and the many micronutrients are essential to life and because most of them cannot be made by the body, we must get these nutrients from food or from nutritional supplements. The U.S. Department of Agriculture (USDA) encourages Americans to eat a well-balanced diet, which it illustrates with a diagram known as the Food Guide Pyramid. At the base of the pyramid are breads, cereals, rice, and pasta. Six to eleven servings from this group are recommended daily—more servings than from any other group of foods in the pyramid. The next level is occupied by vegetables, with three to five daily servings recommended, and by fruit, with two to four servings recommended. Moving upward, the next level is shared by milk, yogurt, and cheese—two to three servings—and meat, poultry, fish, dry beans, eggs, and nuts—two to three servings. Finally, at the peak of the pyramid are fats, oils, and sweets, for which there are no recommended amounts, only a note that they should be consumed sparingly.

To ensure that you have adequate servings of healthful foods, it is a good idea to follow the Food Guide Pyramid and, within each group, to choose foods that are high in the nutrients needed for good health. The remainder of this book shows how each food rates in terms of its nutrient values.

The following section should provide you with the details you need to better access and understand the data contained in this volume. With this information, and the information that makes up the bulk of this book, you will be equipped to learn more about your unique nutritional needs and the foods you are using to meet those needs. You should enjoy the sense of control this knowledge gives you. More important, you will make better food choices and take a major step toward better health.

FOOD GUIDE PYRAMID
A Guide to Daily Food Choices

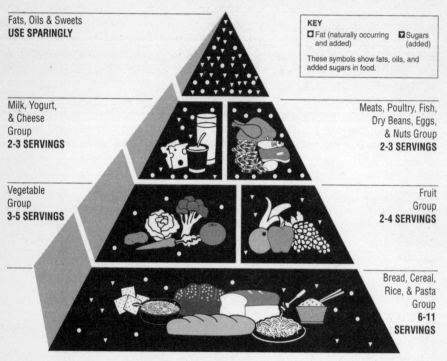

Fats, Oils & Sweets
USE SPARINGLY

KEY
☐ Fat (naturally occurring and added)   ▼ Sugars (added)

These symbols show fats, oils, and added sugars in food.

Milk, Yogurt, & Cheese Group
2-3 SERVINGS

Meats, Poultry, Fish, Dry Beans, Eggs, & Nuts Group
2-3 SERVINGS

Vegetable Group
3-5 SERVINGS

Fruit Group
2-4 SERVINGS

Bread, Cereal, Rice, & Pasta Group
6-11 SERVINGS

Source: U.S. Department of Agriculture & U.S. Department of Health and Human Services

HOW TO USE THIS BOOK

This book was designed to provide comprehensive nutritional information on a wide range of foods. The information provided here was gleaned from a number of government agencies, from hundreds of manufacturers, and from food trade associations. This information was compiled and later supplemented through countless hours of follow-up that involved hundreds of additional sources. Because scientific techniques are continually being improved, this book will be continually updated to reflect the most current nutritional data available.

FINDING THE LISTING YOU WANT

All of the foods in this reference have been listed alphabetically, by restaurant. For convenience, similar foods have sometimes been grouped together in categories such as *Dessert, Sandwich,* and so forth. Therefore, if the food you are looking for is not listed individually by its own name, you should try looking it up under a logical category.

If you are unable to find a particular food, look for the entry for a similar food. The nutritional data should be close, if not exact, for any product not listed.

After you locate the listing for the food you are interested in, you may find that abbreviations have been used to provide you with the information you need. Refer to page xv for a key to the abbreviations used throughout this book.

One feature that sets this book apart from many other nutrition books is the inclusion of the column called "% Fat Calories." Although scientists and nutritionists can use any of several methods to determine the percentage of calories derived from fat, the simplest and most popular is the "4-4-9" method. This technique assumes that 1 gram of protein contains 4 calories, that 1 gram of carbohydrate contains 4 calories, and that 1 gram of fat contains 9 calories. In beverages and foods containing alcohol, it is assumed that each gram of alcohol contains 7 calories. Once you know the total calories and the calories from fat, the calculations used to determine the percentage of calories from fat are, in theory, fairly straightforward and accurate.

When applied to actual published nutrition data, however, several factors make the 4-4-9 method less than ideal. For one thing, many manufacturers consider any nutrient containing fewer than 5 calories to be "nutritionally insignificant." For this reason, the manufacturers round off their published values for protein, carbohydrates, and fats. Sometimes they publish a value of "< 1.0 gram" of fat, which means that the fat content might be anywhere from 0.0 grams to 0.99 grams. When a food item contains only a few calories, the "insignificant" rounding of fat values can have significant and misleading consequences.

One consequence of this practice of rounding off values is that when the calorie values for protein, carbohydrates, and fat are added up, they very rarely match the calorie values published by the manufacturer or restaurant. This means that to simply multiply fat grams by 9 will often result in a misleading value for percentage of calories from fat.

To more accurately represent the percentage of calories from fat, we developed a simple method called the compensated 4-4-9 method. Here is how this method was used to calculate the percentage-of-calories-from-fat values that appear in this book.

1. We calculated the total calories from each of the calorie sources by multiplying protein grams by 4, carbohydrate grams by 4, and fat grams by 9. We added these values together to get a "total derived calories" value.
2. We made the assumption that the manufacturer's total calorie value was correct. We then compared our total derived calorie value to the manufacturer's published total calorie value. If our derived value was lower or higher, we adjusted all of the nonzero nutrient values—maintaining the 4-4-9 ratio—to match the manufacturer's total.
3. Using the adjusted nutrient values, we calculated the percentage of calories from fat.

The compensated 4-4-9 method results in percentage-of-calories values for protein, carbohydrates, and fats that both match the manufacturer's calorie figure for each nutrient and add up to 100 percent of the total calories. Using the nutritional information provided by the manufacturers at this time, we feel that this method is the best means of determining accurate values.

CODES AND ABBREVIATIONS

To provide the most comprehensive nutritional information possible, a number of codes and abbreviations have been used throughout this book. A complete translation is given below.

>	greater than		nia	niacin
<	less than		pkg	package
approx	approximately		pot	potassium
cal	calories		prep	prepared according to directions
calc	calcium		prot	protein
carbs	carbohydrates		rib	riboflavin
fl	fluid		sat fat	saturated fat
fol	folic acid		sod	sodium
gm	gram		tbsp	tablespoon
IU	international unit[1]		thi	thiamine
lb	pound		tr	trace
mag	magnesium		(tr)	may contain a trace amount
mcg	microgram(s)		tsp	teaspoon
med	medium-sized		w/	with
mg	milligram(s)		w/o	without
(mq)	may contain a measurable quantity[2]		wt	weight
na	not available		zn	zinc

[1] International units, which are used throughout this book to express vitamin A content, are a measure of fat-soluble vitamin activity. The amounts of all other nutrients are expressed in grams or milligrams, which are units of mass and weight.

[2] The food item may contain a quantity ranging from a trace amount to a substantial amount. This quantity depends upon any one of a number of variables—such as soil condition and mineral content of fertilizer used—that may have affected the food item during growing, processing, and/or preparation.

Fast-Food/Chain
Restaurant Values

Food Name	Serv. Size	Total Cal.	Prot. gms	Carbs gms	Sod. mgs	Fiber gms	Fat gms	Chol. mgs	Sat.Fat gms	%Fat Cal.
ARBY'S										
BACON	2 strips	90	5	0	220	0	7.0	10.0	3	76%
BISCUIT										
w/margarine	2.8 oz	270	5	26	750	0	16.0	0.0	3	54%
CATSUP/KETCHUP	1 pkt	10	na	3	90	0	0.0	0.0	0	0%
CHEESE										
Swiss	1 slice	45	3	0	220	0	3.0	10.0	2	69%
CROISSANT	2.2 oz	260	6	28	300	0	16.0	20.0	10	51%
DRESSING										
bleu cheese	2.5 oz	390	3	3	770	0	39.0	30.0	6	94%
buttermilk ranch	2.5 oz	210	0	2	600	0	49.0	5.0	7	98%
buttermilk ranch, reduced calorie	2 oz	50	0	12	710	0	0.0	0.0	0	0%
honey French	2.5 oz	350	0	24	530	0	27.0	0.0	4	72%
Italian, lower calorie	2.19 oz	20	0	4	1110	0	1.0	0.0	0	36%
Thousand Island	2.5 oz	350	0	11	580	0	33.0	15.0	5	87%
EGG										
scrambled	1.8 oz	70	6	0	70	0	5.0	220.0	2	65%
FINGER MEAL										
chicken	10.7 oz	880	35	81	2240	0	47.0	60.0	8	48%
FINGER SNACK										
chicken	7.4 oz	610	20	62	1610	0	32.0	30.0	6	47%
jalapeño bites	3.9 oz	330	7	29	670	2	21.0	40.0	9	57%
mozzarella sticks	4.8 oz	470	18	34	1330	2	29.0	60.0	14	56%
onion petals	4 oz	410	4	43	300	2	24.0	0.0	3	53%
FRENCH FRIES										
cheddar curly	6 oz	450	8	52	1420	0	25.0	5.0	6	49%
curly, large	7 oz	600	8	75	1710	0	30.0	0.0	7	45%
curly, medium	4.5 oz	380	5	49	1100	0	19.0	0.0	5	44%
curly, small	3.8 oz	320	4	40	910	0	16.0	0.0	4	45%
homestyle, large	7.5 oz	630	8	86	1240	6	29.0	0.0	5	41%
homestyle, medium	5 oz	420	5	57	830	4	19.0	0.0	3	41%
homestyle, small	4 oz	340	4	46	660	3	15.0	0.0	3	40%
FRENCH TOASTIX, w/o powdered										
sugar or syrup	3 hotcakes	370	7	48	440	4	17.0	0.0	4	41%
HAM	1.5 oz	50	7	1	830	0	3.0	30.0	1	46%
HOT CHOCOLATE	8.6 oz	110	2	23	120	0	1.0	0.0	1	8%
MAPLE SYRUP	1.5 oz	220	0	54	50	0	0.0	0.0	0	0%
MUSTARD										
German	1 pkt	5	0	0	60	0	0.0	0.0	0	0%
honey	1 oz	130	0	5	170	0	12.0	10.0	2	84%
ORANGE JUICE	10 oz	140	1	34	0	0	0.0	0.0	0	0%
POTATO, BAKED										
broccoli 'n cheddar	13.6 oz	550	14	71	730	7	25.0	50.0	13	40%
chicken broccoli	15.8 oz	830	35	68	970	7	47.0	60.0	8	51%
cool ranch	12.3 oz	500	8	67	150	6	23.0	25.0	7	41%
deluxe	12.3 oz	610	14	68	860	6	31.0	80.0	19	46%
jalapeño	14.6 oz	660	15	72	930	6	36.0	50.0	14	48%

Food Name	Serv. Size	Total Cal.	Prot. gms	Carbs gms	Sod. mgs	Fiber gms	Fat gms	Chol. mgs	Sat.Fat gms	%Fat Cal.
Philly chicken	15.8 oz	880	32	75	1020	7	53.0	70.0	10	53%
w/butter and sour cream	11.3 oz	500	8	65	170	6	24.0	60.0	15	43%
POTATO CAKES	2 cakes	220	2	21	460	3	14.0	0.0	3	58%
SALAD										
garden, w/one crouton packet, 2 saltine crackers	10.2 oz	110	9	16	150	1	3.0	0.0	0	21%
grilled chicken, low-fat	14.2 oz	190	25	16	530	1	4.0	40.0	1	18%
roast chicken, lowfat	14.2 oz	200	25	16	800	1	5.0	40.0	1	22%
w/one crouton packet, 2 saltine crackers	5.4 oz	90	5	12	130	0	3.0	0.0	0	28%
SANDWICH										
Arby-Q	6.6 oz	380	19	42	990	3	15.0	30.0	5	36%
Beef 'N Cheddar	7 oz	510	26	45	1250	3	28.0	50.0	9	47%
chicken, bacon 'n Swiss	7.8 oz	610	37	52	1620	5	30.0	75.0	9	43%
chicken breast fillet	7.6 oz	560	30	49	1080	6	28.0	55.0	6	44%
chicken cordon bleu	8.9 oz	650	40	50	2120	5	34.0	90.0	9	46%
fish fillet sandwich	7.9 oz	540	23	51	880	2	27.0	40.0	7	45%
French dip sub	7.1 oz	490	30	43	1440	3	22.0	56.0	8	40%
grilled chicken, lowfat	6.3 oz	280	30	33	920	4	5.0	50.0	2	15%
grilled chicken deluxe	8.7 oz	420	30	42	930	3	16.0	60.0	4	33%
hot ham 'n Swiss sub	9.7 oz	570	30	47	2660	2	31.0	100.0	10	48%
Italian sub.	10.3 oz	800	28	49	2610	2	54.0	85.0	16	61%
Philly beef 'n Swiss sub	11.1 oz	780	39	52	2140	4	48.0	90.0	16	54%
roast beef, big Montana	11 oz	720	50	44	2270	7	40.0	110.0	17	49%
roast beef, giant.	8.1 oz	550	34	43	1560	5	28.0	70.0	11	45%
roast beef, junior.	4.6 oz	340	18	36	790	3	16.0	30.0	6	40%
roast beef, regular.	5.6 oz	400	23	36	1030	3	20.0	40.0	7	43%
roast beef, super.	8.7 oz	530	24	50	1190	5	27.0	40.0	9	45%
roast beef melt w/cheddar.	5.4 oz	380	19	38	960	3	19.0	30.0	7	43%
roast beef sub.	10.7 oz	770	32	48	2170	3	49.0	70.0	15	58%
roast chicken club.	8.4 oz	540	37	39	1590	3	29.0	70.0	8	46%
roast chicken deluxe, low-fat.	7 oz	260	23	32	950	4	5.0	40.0	2	17%
roast turkey deluxe, lowfat.	6.9 oz	230	19	33	870	4	5.0	25.0	2	18%
turkey sub	10.7 oz	670	29	49	2130	2	39.0	60.0	10	53%
SAUCE										
Arby's	1 pkt	15	0	3	110	0	0.0	0.0	0	0%
barbecue dipping	1 oz	40	0	10	350	0	0.0	0.0	0	0%
beef stock au jus	2 oz	10	0	0	440	0	0.0	0.0	0	0%
bronco berry	1.5 oz	90	0	23	35	0	0.0	0.0	0	0%
horsey	1 pkt	60	0	3	100	0	5.0	0.0	1	79%
marinara sauce	1.5 oz	35	1	4	260	0	1.5	0.0	0	40%
tangy Southwest	1.52 oz	250	0	3	280	0	25.0	30.0	4	95%
SAUSAGE PATTY	1.4 oz	200	7	1	290	0	19.0	60.0	7	84%
SHAKE										
chocolate	10.3 oz	390	8	69	270	0	9.0	10.0	6	21%
jamocha	10.3 oz	380	8	66	300	0	9.0	10.0	6	21%
strawberry	10.3 oz	380	8	67	270	0	9.0	10.0	6	21%
vanilla	10.3 oz	380	8	67	270	0	9.0	12.0	6	21%

Food Name	Serv. Size	Total Cal.	Prot. gms	Carbs gms	Sod. mgs	Fiber gms	Fat gms	Chol. mgs	Sat.Fat gms	%Fat Cal.
TURNOVER										
iced apple	3.4 oz	360	4	54	180	6	14.0	0.0	3	35%
iced cherry	3.5 oz	350	4	53	190	0	14.0	0.0	3	36%
ARTHUR TREACHER'S										
CHICKEN PATTIES										
	2 patties	369	27	17	495	0	21.6	65.0	4	53%
COD FILLET, 'Bake'n Broil' tail shape	5 oz	245	20	10	144	0	14.2	0.0	0	52%
COLESLAW										
	3 oz	123	1	11	266	0	8.2	7.0	1	60%
DESSERT, Lemon Luv	1 serving	276	3	35	314	0	13.9	1.0	2	45%
FISH FILLET	5.2 oz	355	19	25	450	0	19.8	56.0	3	50%
FRENCH FRIES, chips	4 oz	276	4	35	39	0	13.2	5.0	2	43%
HUSHPUPPY, 'Krunch Pup'	1 piece	203	5	12	446	0	14.8	25.0	4	66%
SANDWICH										
chicken	1 sandwich	413	16	44	708	0	19.2	32.0	3	42%
fish	1 sandwich	440	16	39	836	0	24.0	42.0	4	49%
SHRIMP	7 pieces	381	13	27	538	0	24.4	93.0	3	58%
AU BON PAIN										
BAGEL										
cinnamon	1 bagel	395	14	86	605	4	2.0	0.0	1	4%
onion	1 bagel	390	16	81	665	4	2.0	0.0	1	4%
plain	1 bagel	380	15	79	665	3	2.0	0.0	1	5%
sesame	1 bagel	425	17	81	665	4	5.0	0.0	1	10%
BREAD										
baguette	1 loaf	810	27	166	1830	0	2.0	0.0	1	2%
cheese	1 loaf	1670	70	269	4140	0	29.0	75.0	9	16%
four-grain	1 loaf	1420	57	262	3050	0	11.0	1.0	1	7%
multigrain	2 slices	391	16	77	2040	0	3.0	1.0	1	7%
onion herb	1 loaf	1430	52	263	2390	0	13.0	0.0	1	9%
pita pocket	2 slices	80	3	18	0	0	1.0	0.0	0	10%
ponsienne	1 loaf	1490	49	166	3380	0	4.0	0.0	1	4%
rye	2 slices	374	14	73	2170	0	4.0	0.0	1	9%
CHICKEN POT PIE	1 serving	440	18	46	1109	0	21.0	45.0	7	43%
COOKIE										
chocolate chip	1 cookie	280	2	37	70	0	15.0	25.0	9	46%
chocolate chunk, w/pecan, 'Gourmet'	1 cookie	290	3	37	200	0	17.0	10.0	6	49%
cookie, oatmeal, oatmeal raisin, 'Gourmet'	1 cookie	250	4	41	230	0	9.0	10.0	0	31%
peanut butter, 'Gourmet'	1 cookie	290	7	33	250	0	15.0	10.0	6	46%
shortbread, 'Gourmet'	1 cookie	425	5	46	385	0	26.0	68.0	16	53%
white chocolate chunk, w/pecan, 'Gourmet'	1 cookie	300	3	37	200	0	17.0	10.0	6	49%
CROISSANT										
almond	1 croissant	420	8	41	250	0	25.0	95.0	12	53%
apple	1 croissant	250	4	38	150	0	10.0	25.0	6	35%
blueberry cheese	1 croissant	380	7	44	280	0	20.0	60.0	12	47%
chocolate	1 croissant	400	5	46	220	0	24.0	35.0	14	51%

Food Name	Serv. Size	Total Cal.	Prot. gms	Carbs gms	Sod. mgs	Fiber gms	Fat gms	Chol. mgs	Sat.Fat gms	%Fat Cal.
cinnamon raisin	1 croissant	390	7	60	240	0	13.0	35.0	8	30%
coconut pecan	1 croissant	440	7	51	290	0	23.0	45.0	12	47%
croissant, plain	1 croissant	220	5	29	240	0	10.0	25.0	6	40%
hazelnut chocolate	1 croissant	480	6	56	220	0	28.0	35.0	14	50%
raspberry cheese	1 croissant	400	7	49	280	0	20.0	60.0	12	45%
strawberry cheese	1 croissant	400	7	49	280	0	20.0	60.0	12	45%
sweet cheese	1 croissant	420	8	45	310	0	23.0	70.0	14	49%
MUFFIN										
blueberry, gourmet	1 muffin	390	8	66	410	0	4.0	40.0	0	11%
bran, gourmet	1 muffin	390	7	73	940	0	11.0	20.0	0	24%
carrot, gourmet	1 muffin	450	7	58	610	0	22.0	15.0	5	43%
corn, gourmet	1 muffin	460	8	71	510	0	17.0	25.0	3	33%
cranberry walnut, gourmet	1 muffin	350	7	53	730	0	13.0	15.0	0	33%
oat bran apple gourmet	1 muffin	400	7	71	590	0	2.0	0.0	0	5%
pumpkin gourmet	1 muffin	410	6	63	500	0	16.0	20.0	2	34%
whole grain, gourmet	1 muffin	440	10	68	310	0	16.0	30.0	2	32%
PASTRY										
cheese Danish	1 Danish	390	8	43	530	2	22.0	78.0	12	49%
cherry Danish	1 Danish	335	7	42	480	2	16.0	50.0	8	42%
cherry dumpling Danish	1 Danish	360	5	59	255	1	13.0	0.0	2	31%
raspberry Danish	1 Danish	335	6	43	480	2	16.0	50.0	8	42%
ROLL										
'Alpine'	1 roll	220	8	43	810	0	3.0	0.0	0	12%
braided	1 roll	387	10	64	1540	0	11.0	34.0	3	25%
country seed	1 roll	220	9	37	460	0	4.0	0.0	0	16%
croissant	1 roll	300	7	38	240	0	14.0	35.0	8	41%
French	1 roll	320	10	65	710	0	1.0	0.0	0	3%
hearth	1 roll	370	16	69	600	0	3.0	0.0	0	7%
'Petit Pain'	1 roll	220	7	44	490	0	1.0	0.0	0	4%
pumpernickel	1 roll	210	8	42	1005	0	2.0	0.0	0	8%
raisin	1 roll	250	8	46	480	0	4.0	0.0	0	14%
rye	1 roll	230	8	44	0	0	2.0	0.0	0	8%
soft	1 roll	310	8	50	410	0	8.0	0.0	0	24%
vegetable	1 roll	230	6	40	410	0	5.0	0.0	0	20%
SALAD										
garden, small	1 salad	20	5	5	10	0	1.0	0.0	0	18%
garden w/grilled chicken	1 salad	110	14	9	330	0	2.0	30.0	0	16%
garden w/shrimp	1 salad	102	11	8	193	0	2.0	105.0	0	19%
garden w/tuna	1 salad	350	21	11	480	0	25.0	40.0	4	64%
Italian, low-calorie	1 salad	68	0	3	360	0	6.0	5.0	0	82%
SANDWICH										
chicken, cracked pepper, on French roll	1 sandwich	440	33	66	1390	0	3.0	50.0	0	6%
chicken, cracked pepper, on hearth roll	1 sandwich	490	39	70	1280	0	5.0	50.0	0	9%
chicken, cracked pepper, on soft roll	1 sandwich	430	31	51	1090	0	10.0	50.0	0	22%
chicken, grilled, on French roll	1 sandwich	450	33	66	1320	0	5.0	60.0	0	10%
chicken, grilled, on hearth roll	1 sandwich	500	39	70	1210	0	7.0	60.0	0	13%
chicken, grilled, on soft roll	1 sandwich	440	31	51	1020	0	12.0	60.0	0	25%
chicken, tarragon, on French roll	1 sandwich	590	34	68	1014	0	16.0	70.0	0	26%

Food Name	Serv. Size	Total Cal.	Prot. gms	Carbs gms	Sod. mgs	Fiber gms	Fat gms	Chol. mgs	Sat.Fat gms	%Fat Cal.
chicken, tarragon, on hearth roll	1 sandwich	640	40	72	904	0	18.0	70.0	0	27%
chicken, tarragon, on soft roll	1 sandwich	580	32	53	714	0	23.0	70.0	0	38%
ham, on French roll	1 sandwich	470	27	68	1680	0	8.0	115.0	0	16%
ham, on hearth roll	1 sandwich	520	33	72	1570	0	10.0	115.0	0	18%
ham, on soft roll	1 sandwich	460	25	53	1380	0	15.0	115.0	0	30%
ham and cheese croissant, hot, filled	1 sandwich	370	10	38	280	0	20.0	55.0	12	48%
roast beef, on French roll	1 sandwich	500	34	66	1020	0	9.0	60.0	0	17%
roast beef, on hearth roll	1 sandwich	550	40	70	910	0	11.0	60.0	0	18%
roast beef, on soft roll	1 sandwich	490	32	51	720	0	16.0	60.0	0	30%
spinach and cheese croissant, hot, filled	1 sandwich	290	9	29	310	0	16.0	45.0	10	49%
turkey and cheddar croissant, hot, filled	1 sandwich	410	16	38	680	0	22.0	70.0	13	48%
turkey and havarti croissant, hot, filled	1 sandwich	410	17	38	630	0	21.0	70.0	13	46%
turkey sandwich, smoked, on French roll	1 sandwich	420	32	65	1660	0	2.0	35.0	0	4%
turkey sandwich, smoked, on hearth roll	1 sandwich	470	38	69	1550	0	4.0	35.0	0	8%
turkey sandwich, smoked, on soft roll	1 sandwich	410	30	50	1360	0	9.0	35.0	0	20%
SANDWICH FILLING										
boursin cheese	1 serving	290	6	2	390	0	29.0	90.0	18	89%
brie cheese	1 serving	300	18	3	510	0	24.0	85.0	15	72%
provolone cheese	1 serving	155	10	1	180	0	12.6	36.0	7	72%
SOUP										
beef barley	1 bowl	112	9	15	901	0	3.0	18.0	0	22%
beef barley	1 cup	75	6	10	600	0	2.0	12.0	0	22%
broccoli, cream of	1 bowl	302	8	18	219	0	26.0	54.0	12	69%
broccoli, cream of	1 cup	201	5	12	146	0	17.0	36.0	8	69%
chicken, w/noodle	1 bowl	119	12	14	743	0	1.7	26.0	1	13%
chicken, w/noodle................	1 cup	79	8	9	495	0	1.0	17.0	1	12%
chili, vegetarian	1 bowl	208	9	37	763	0	4.0	0.0	1	16%
chili, vegetarian	1 cup	139	6	24	508	0	3.0	0.0	1	18%
clam chowder	1 bowl	433	17	36	1029	0	27.0	90.0	15	53%
clam chowder....................	1 cup	289	11	24	687	0	18.0	60.0	9	54%
minestrone......................	1 cup	105	5	20	265	0	2.0	1.0	0	15%
split pea........................	1 bowl	264	18	45	453	0	2.0	1.0	0	7%
split pea........................	1 cup	176	12	30	303	0	1.0	1.0	0	5%
tomato Florentine	1 bowl	92	4	15	221	0	1.7	0.0	1	17%
tomato Florentine	1 cup	61	3	10	147	0	1.0	0.0	1	15%
vegetarian, garden	1 bowl	44	2	9	92	0	1.0	0.0	1	17%
vegetarian, garden...............	1 cup	29	1	6	61	0	1.0	0.0	1	24%

BASKIN-ROBBINS

ICE

Food Name	Serv. Size	Total Cal.	Prot. gms	Carbs gms	Sod. mgs	Fiber gms	Fat gms	Chol. mgs	Sat.Fat gms	%Fat Cal.
grape	1/2 cup	100	0	27	10	0	0.0	0.0	0	0%
margarita.......................	1/2 cup	110	0	28	10	0	0.0	0.0	0	0%
ICE CREAM										
'Berries 'n Banana,' sugarless	1/2 cup	80	4	15	55	0	1.0	5.0	1	11%

Food Name	Serv. Size	Total Cal.	Prot. gms	Carbs gms	Sod. mgs	Fiber gms	Fat gms	Chol. mgs	Sat.Fat gms	%Fat Cal.
'Call Me Nuts,' sugarless	1/2 cup	110	3	21	55	1	2.0	5.0	1	16%
'Cappuccino Blast,' w/whipped cream	1 serving	160	3	22	60	0	7.0	30.0	4	39%
'Caramel Banana Surprise,' nonfat	1/2 cup	110	3	24	95	0	0.0	0.0	0	0%
caramel praline, soft serve, nonfat	1/2 cup	120	4	25	85	0	0.0	0.0	0	0%
'Cherry Cordial,' sugarless	1/2 cup	100	3	18	55	0	2.0	5.0	2	18%
chocolate chip, 'Chillyburger'	1 serving	220	4	27	100	1	11.0	25.0	7	44%
chocolate chip, sugarless	1/2 cup	100	4	17	70	0	2.5	5.5	2	21%
chocolate chip, sugarless, 'Low, Lite 'n Luscious'	1 serving	100	3	20	0	0	2.0	4.0	0	16%
chocolate marshmallow, nonfat	1/2 cup	110	4	26	75	1	0.0	0.0	0	0%
chocolate vanilla twist, nonfat	1/2 cup	100	4	21	100	0	0.0	0.0	0	0%
'Chocolate Wonder,' nonfat.	1/2 cup	90	4	20	70	1	0.0	0.0	0	0%
'Chunky Banana,' sugarless	1/2 cup	90	3	16	55	0	1.5	5.0	1	15%
coconut fudge, sugarless	1/2 cup	110	3	20	60	1	1.5	5.0	1	13%
'Double Raspberry,' light	1/2 cup	90	3	16	40	0	2.0	10.0	1	19%
espresso, light	1/2 cup	110	3	18	55	0	4.0	10.0	3	30%
'Jamoca Swirl,' nonfat	1/2 cup	110	3	23	105	0	0.0	0.0	0	0%
'Jamoca Swiss Almond,' sugarless	1/2 cup	100	3	16	65	0	2.5	5.0	2	23%
'Just Chocolate Vanilla' dairy, nonfat	1/2 cup	100	4	21	60	0	0.0	0.0	0	0%
'Just Peachy' dairy, nonfat	1/2 cup	100	3	22	60	0	0.0	0.0	0	0%
'Kookaberry Kiwi,' nonfat.	1/2 cup	90	3	20	90	0	0.0	0.0	0	0%
'Mocha Cappuccino Blast,' nonfat	1 serving	120	3	26	75	0	0.0	0.0	0	0%
peach, nonfat.	1/2 cup	100	3	22	90	0	0.0	0.0	0	0%
peanut butter cream, nonfat.	1/2 cup	100	4	21	110	0	0.0	0.0	0	0%
pineapple cheesecake, nonfat.	1/2 cup	110	3	24	100	0	0.0	0.0	0	0%
pineapple coconut, sugarless.	1/2 cup	90	3	16	60	0	1.5	5.0	1	15%
'Pistachio Creme Chip,' light.	1/2 cup	120	4	17	55	0	4.0	10.0	3	30%
'Pralines 'n Cream'	1 scoop	280	4	35	180	0	14.0	36.0	0	45%
praline, light.	1/2 cup	120	3	18	65	0	4.0	10.0	2	30%
'Raspberry Revelation' sugarless	1/2 cup	100	3	20	55	1	1.0	5.0	1	9%
'Rocky Path,' light.	1/2 cup	130	4	19	55	1	4.0	10.0	2	28%
strawberry, sugarless, 'Low, Lite 'n Luscious'	1 serving	80	2	17	70	0	1.0	3.0	0	11%
'Strawberry Royal,' light	1/2 cup	110	2	19	120	0	3.0	9.0	0	24%
vanilla, soft serve, nonfat.	1/2 cup	120	5	25	85	0	0.0	0.0	0	0%
'Thin Mint,' sugarless.	1/2 cup	100	3	16	65	0	2.5	5.0	2	23%
'Vanilla Bean,' nonfat.	1/2 cup	100	4	20	110	0	0.0	0.0	0	0%
'Vanilla Swiss Almond,' sugarless	1/2 cup	110	3	20	60	1	2.0	5.0	2	16%
ICE CREAM BAR										
'Sundae Bars' chocolate, caramel ribbon, light	1 bar	150	3	24	75	0	5.0	11.0	0	29%
'Cappuccino Blast'	1 bar	120	2	18	35	0	5.0	20.0	3	36%
ICE CREAM CONE										
waffle, cone and cup, plain	1 cone	140	3	28	5	0	2.0	0.0	0	13%
sugar, cone and cup, plain	1 cone	60	1	11	45	0	1.0	0.0	0	16%
SHERBET										
orange	1/2 cup	120	1	26	25	0	1.5	5.0	1	11%
rainbow	1/2 cup	120	1	26	25	0	1.5	5.0	1	11%

Food Name	Serv. Size	Total Cal.	Prot. gms	Carbs gms	Sod. mgs	Fiber gms	Fat gms	Chol. mgs	Sat.Fat gms	%Fat Cal.
SORBET										
fruit whip, nonfat	1 serving	80	0	24	20	0	0.0	0.0	0	0%
raspberry cranberry	1/2 cup	110	0	29	10	0	0.0	0.0	0	0%
red raspberry	1/2 cup	120	0	30	10	0	0.0	0.0	0	0%
strawberry, soft-serve, nonfat	1 serving	100	0	20	20	0	0.0	0.0	0	0%
TOPPING										
butterscotch	1 oz	100	1	24	80	0	1.0	3.0	1	9%
hot fudge	1 oz	100	1	17	45	0	3.0	0.0	1	27%
hot fudge, nonfat, sugar-free	1 oz	90	2	20	96	1	0.0	0.0	0	0%
praline caramel	1 oz	90	0	19	105	0	0.0	0.0	0	0%
strawberry	1 oz	60	0	14	5	0	0.0	0.0	0	0%
YOGURT, FROZEN										
black cherry, nonfat	1/2 cup	110	3	24	50	0	0.0	0.0	0	0%
blueberry, lowfat	1/2 cup	120	4	24	70	0	1.5	5.0	1	11%
cheesecake, lowfat	1/2 cup	120	4	21	75	0	1.5	10.0	1	12%
chocolate, lowfat	1/2 cup	120	5	23	75	0	1.5	5.0	1	11%
chocolate, lowfat, large	9 oz	315	9	54	90	0	9.0	9.0	0	24%
chocolate, lowfat, medium	7 oz	246	7	42	70	0	7.0	7.0	0	24%
chocolate mint, nonfat	1/2 cup	100	4	23	60	1	0.0	0.0	0	0%
coconut, nonfat, large	9 oz	180	9	45	90	0	0.0	0.0	0	0%
coconut, nonfat, medium	7 oz	140	7	35	70	0	0.0	0.0	0	0%
coconut, nonfat, small	5 oz	100	5	25	50	0	0.0	0.0	0	0%
Dutch chocolate, nonfat	1/2 cup	100	4	23	60	1	0.0	0.0	0	0%
'For Heaven's Cake,' low-fat	1/2 cup	120	3	24	75	0	2.0	10.0	2	14%
'Have Your Cake,' low-fat	1/2 cup	110	4	22	100	0	1.0	4.0	1	8%
Kahlua frozen, nonfat	1/2 cup	100	3	21	55	0	0.0	0.0	0	0%
key lime nonfat.	1/2 cup	100	3	22	55	0	0.0	0.0	0	0%
'Mango in Paradise,' nonfat.	1/2 cup	130	4	28	70	1	0.0	0.0	0	0%
maple walnut, nonfat.	1/2 cup	100	3	22	55	0	0.0	0.0	0	0%
peach, nonfat.	1/2 cup	100	3	22	50	0	0.0	0.0	0	0%
'Peppermint Twist,' nonfat.	1/2 cup	100	3	22	55	0	0.0	0.0	0	0%
piña colada, nonfat.	1/2 cup	110	3	22	50	0	0.0	0.0	0	0%
raspberry, nonfat.	1/2 cup	100	3	22	55	0	0.0	0.0	0	0%
raspberry, nonfat, large	9 oz	225	9	45	90	0	0.0	0.0	0	0%
raspberry, nonfat, medium	7 oz	164	7	35	70	0	0.0	0.0	0	0%
raspberry, nonfat, small	5 oz	125	5	25	50	0	0.0	0.0	0	0%
strawberry, low-fat, large	9 oz	270	9	54	90	0	9.0	9.0	0	24%
strawberry, low-fat, medium	7 oz	211	7	42	70	0	7.0	7.0	0	24%
strawberry, low-fat, small	5 oz	150	5	30	50	0	5.0	5.0	0	24%
strawberry, nonfat.	1/2 cup	100	3	23	55	0	0.0	0.0	0	0%
strawberry, nonfat, large.	9 oz	225	9	45	90	0	0.0	0.0	0	0%
strawberry, nonfat, medium	7 oz	176	7	35	70	0	0.0	0.0	0	0%
vanilla, low-fat	1/2 cup	120	4	22	75	0	2.0	10.0	1	15%
vanilla, low-fat, large	9 oz	270	9	54	90	0	9.0	9.0	0	24%
vanilla, low-fat, medium	7 oz	211	7	42	70	0	7.0	7.0	0	24%
vanilla, nonfat	1/2 cup	110	4	23	65	0	0.0	0.0	0	0%

BIG BOY RESTAURANT

Food Name	Serv. Size	Total Cal.	Prot. gms	Carbs gms	Sod. mgs	Fiber gms	Fat gms	Chol. mgs	Sat.Fat gms	%Fat Cal.
DESSERT										
'No-no' frozen	1 serving	75	2	17	36	0	0.0	0.0	0	0%

Food Name	Serv. Size	Total Cal.	Prot. gms	Carbs gms	Sod. mgs	Fiber gms	Fat gms	Chol. mgs	Sat.Fat gms	%Fat Cal.
yogurt, frozen, nonfat	1 serving	72	2	16	31	0	0.0	0.0	0	0%
ENTRÉE										
chicken and vegetable stir-fry	1 serving	562	43	68	750	0	14.0	68.0	0	22%
chicken breast, w/salad, no dressing, oat bran bread	1 serving	349	38	20	342	0	13.0	65.0	0	34%
chicken breast, w/mozzarella, salad, no dressing, bread	1 serving	370	42	24	353	0	12.0	76.0	0	29%
chicken, Cajun, w/salad, no dressing, oat bran bread	1 serving	349	38	20	612	0	13.0	65.0	0	34%
cod, baked, w/salad, no dressing, oat bran bread	1 serving	364	43	20	371	0	12.0	68.0	0	30%
cod, broiled, w/salad, no dressing, oat bran bread	1 serving	364	43	20	371	0	12.0	68.0	0	30%
cod, Cajun, w/salad, no dressing, oat bran bread	1 serving	364	43	20	461	0	12.0	68.0	0	30%
cod, Dijon, baked, w/salad, no dressing, bread	1 serving	427	44	21	567	0	18.0	68.0	0	38%
cod, Dijon, broiled, w/salad, no dressing, bread	1 serving	427	44	21	567	0	18.0	68.0	0	38%
spaghetti marinara, w/salad, no dressing, oat bran bread	1 serving	450	15	87	761	0	6.0	8.0	0	12%
vegetable stir-fry	1 serving	408	9	74	703	0	10.0	0.0	0	21%
SALAD										
chicken breast, Dijon	1 salad	391	42	31	415	0	11.0	65.0	0	25%
dinner, no dressing	1 salad	19	1	4	11	0	0.0	0.0	0	0%
SALAD DRESSING, buttermilk	1 serving	36	0	4	151	0	2.0	10.0	0	53%
SANDWICH										
chicken w/mozzarella, on pita, 'Heart Smart'	1 sandwich	404	42	26	421	0	13.0	76.0	0	30%
turkey, on pita, 'Heart Smart'	1 sandwich	224	22	24	833	0	5.0	75.0	0	20%
SIDE DISH										
corn	1 serving	90	3	21	1	0	1.0	0.0	0	9%
mixed vegetables	1 serving	27	2	5	42	0	0.0	0.0	0	0%
potato, baked	1 serving	163	5	37	7	0	0.0	0.0	0	0%
rice	1 serving	114	3	25	633	0	0.0	0.0	0	0%
roll	1 roll	139	3	30	187	0	0.0	2.0	0	0%
SOUP										
cabbage	1 bowl	43	2	9	727	0	1.0	1.0	0	17%
cabbage	1 cup	37	2	8	623	0	0.0	1.0	0	0%
BOJANGLES										
BISCUIT	1 serving	239	4	30	588	0	11.0	1.0	0	42%
CHICKEN										
breast, no skin, 'Southern'	3.5 oz	239	25	10	766	0	11.5	91.7	0	43%
breast, no skin, 'Southern'	4 oz	271	28	11	869	0	13.0	104.0	0	43%
leg, no skin, 'Southern'	1.8 oz	128	7	5	312	0	12.0	54.0	0	69%
leg, no skin, 'Southern'	3.5 oz	251	14	10	611	0	23.5	105.8	0	69%
thigh, no skin, 'Southern'	3.5 oz	291	21	11	653	0	18.7	97.0	0	57%
thigh, no skin, 'Southern'	3.2 oz	264	19	10	592	0	17.0	88.0	0	57%

Food Name	Serv. Size	Total Cal.	Prot. gms	Carbs gms	Sod. mgs	Fiber gms	Fat gms	Chol. mgs	Sat.Fat gms	%Fat Cal.
SANDWICH, chicken fillet, grilled,										
no mayo	1 sandwich	329	27	37	418	0	7.0	59.0	0	20%
SIDE DISH										
coleslaw	1 serving	105	1	19	406	0	4.0	0.0	0	31%
dirty rice	1 serving	167	5	21	397	0	7.0	12.0	0	38%
pinto bean, Cajun.	1 serving	124	6	25	463	0	0.0	0.0	0	0%

BONANZA RESTAURANTS
HALIBUT FILLET

Food Name	Serv. Size	Total Cal.	Prot. gms	Carbs gms	Sod. mgs	Fiber gms	Fat gms	Chol. mgs	Sat.Fat gms	%Fat Cal.
	6 oz	139	26	3	128	0	2.0	60.0	0	13%
	3.5 oz	82	15	2	75	0	1.2	35.3	0	13%
RIBEYE STEAK										
	5.5 oz	196	28	1	563	0	8.0	50.0	0	38%
	3.5 oz	126	18	1	361	0	5.1	32.1	0	38%

BOSTON MARKET
CHICKEN

Food Name	Serv. Size	Total Cal.	Prot. gms	Carbs gms	Sod. mgs	Fiber gms	Fat gms	Chol. mgs	Sat.Fat gms	%Fat Cal.
drumstick, Tabasco barbecue.	1 drumstick	130	14	4	190	0	6.0	50.0	2	43%
1/4 chicken, dark meat, w/o skin.	1/4 chicken	190	22	1	440	0	10.0	115.0	3	49%
1/4 chicken, dark meat, w/skin.	1/4 chicken	320	30	2	500	0	21.0	155.0	6	60%
1/4 chicken, teriyaki, dark meat, w/skin.	1/4 chicken	380	30	17	870	0	21.0	155.0	6	50%
1/4 chicken, w/skin	1/4 chicken	590	70	4	1010	0	33.0	280.0	10	50%
1/4 chicken, w/wing, white meat, w/skin.	1/4 chicken	280	0	2	510	0	12.0	135.0	4	93%
1/4 chicken, w/o wing, white meat, w/o skin	1/4 chicken	170	33	2	480	0	4.0	85.0	1	20%
Southwest, savory	1 portion	400	40	26	1670	4	15.0	100.0	5	34%
triple topped.	1 portion	470	50	20	1350	1	22.0	155.0	12	41%
wing, Tabasco barbecue.	1 wing	110	9	4	170	0	7.0	30.0	2	55%
CHICKEN POT PIE.	1 pie	780	32	61	1480	4	46.0	135.0	13	53%
CORNBREAD	1 loaf	200	3	33	390	1	6.0	25.0	2	27%
DESSERT										
brownie	1 piece	450	6	47	190	3	27.0	80.0	7	53%
chocolate chip cookie.	1 cookie	340	4	48	240	1	17.0	25.0	6	42%
cinnamon apple pie	1/5 pie	390	2	46	250	2	23.0	0.0	4	52%
GRAVY, chicken.	1 oz	15	0	2	170	0	1.0	0.0	0	53%
HAM, Boston hearth, lean	5 oz	210	25	9	1490	0	9.0	75.0	4	37%
MEAT LOAF										
w/brown gravy	7 oz	390	30	19	1040	1	22.0	120.0	8	50%
w/chunky tomato sauce	8 oz	370	30	22	1170	2	18.0	120.0	8	44%
SALAD										
Caesar, entrée	10 oz	510	17	17	1130	3	42.0	35.0	11	74%
Caesar, side	4 oz	200	7	7	450	1	17.0	15.0	5	73%
Caesar, w/o dressing	8 oz	230	16	14	500	3	12.0	20.0	6	47%
chicken, chunky	3/4 cup	370	28	3	800	1	27.0	120.0	5	66%
chicken Caesar	13 oz	650	43	17	1580	3	45.0	105.0	12	63%
tossed, individual, w/Caesar dressing	1 salad	380	5	18	810	3	31.0	15.0	5	75%

Food Name	Serv. Size	Total Cal.	Prot. gms	Carbs gms	Sod. mgs	Fiber gms	Fat gms	Chol. mgs	Sat.Fat gms	%Fat Cal.
tossed, individual, w/fat-free ranch dressing	1 salad	160	5	29	940	4	2.5	0.0	0	14%
tossed, individual, w/old Venice dressing	1 salad	340	4	20	1110	3	27.0	0.0	4	72%
SANDWICH										
barbecue chicken	1 sandwich	540	30	84	1690	3	9.0	75.0	3	15%
barbecue chicken pastry	1 sandwich	640	17	56	1260	1	39.0	60.0	12	55%
broccoli chicken cheddar pastry	1 sandwich	690	21	45	1050	2	47.0	85.0	13	62%
chicken, w/cheese and sauce sandwich	1 sandwich	750	41	72	1860	5	33.0	135.0	12	40%
chicken, w/o cheese and sauce	1 sandwich	430	34	62	910	4	4.5	65.0	1	10%
chicken salad	1 sandwich	680	39	63	1360	4	30.0	120.0	5	40%
ham, w/cheese and sauce	1 sandwich	750	38	72	1730	5	34.0	100.0	12	41%
ham and cheddar pastry	1 sandwich	640	19	47	1560	1	41.0	60.0	13	58%
ham sub, w/o cheese and sauce	1 sandwich	440	25	66	1450	4	8.0	45.0	3	17%
Italian chicken pastry	1 sandwich	630	21	43	910	2	41.0	60.0	12	59%
meatloaf, w/cheese	1 sandwich	860	46	95	2270	6	33.0	165.0	16	34%
meatloaf, w/o cheese	1 sandwich	690	40	86	1610	6	21.0	120.0	7	27%
turkey, open faced	1 sandwich	500	37	61	2170	3	12.0	80.0	2	22%
turkey, w/cheese and sauce	1 sandwich	710	45	68	1390	4	28.0	110.0	10	36%
turkey club	1 sandwich	650	39	64	1590	4	26.0	105.0	8	36%
turkey sub, w/o cheese and sauce	1 sandwich	400	45	61	1070	4	3.5	60.0	1	7%
SIDE DISH										
applesauce, cinnamon	3/4 cup	250	0	56	45	3	4.5	0.0	1	15%
applesauce, cinnamon, low-fat, chunky	3/4 cup	250	1	62	30	2	0.0	0.0	0	0%
barbecue baked beans	3/4 cup	270	8	48	540	12	5.0	0.0	2	17%
black rice and beans	1 cup	300	8	45	1050	5	10.0	0.0	2	30%
broccoli cauliflower au gratin	3/4 cup	200	9	14	600	3	11.0	20.0	7	52%
broccoli rice casserole	3/4 cup	240	5	26	800	2	12.0	40.0	8	47%
broccoli w/red peppers	3/4 cup	60	3	5	130	3	3.5	0.0	1	50%
butternut squash, low-fat	3/4 cup	160	2	25	580	3	6.0	15.0	4	33%
carrots, honey glazed	3/4 cup	280	1	35	80	4	15.0	0.0	3	48%
chili, chicken	1 cup	220	18	21	1000	6	7.0	40.0	2	29%
coleslaw	3/4 cup	300	2	30	540	3	19.0	20.0	3	57%
corn, whole kernel	3/4 cup	180	5	30	170	2	4.0	0.0	1	20%
coyote bean salad	3/4 cup	190	4	24	210	9	9.0	0.0	1	42%
cranberry relish, low-fat	3/4 cup	370	2	84	5	5	5.0	0.0	1	12%
fruit salad	3/4 cup	70	1	15	10	1	0.5	0.0	0	7%
green beans	3/4 cup	80	1	5	200	3	6.0	0.0	1	69%
green bean casserole	3/4 cup	130	2	10	440	2	9.0	20.0	5	63%
macaroni and cheese	3/4 cup	280	13	32	830	1	11.0	30.0	6	35%
potato, baked, sweet low-fat	1 potato	460	6	94	510	10	7.0	0.0	1	14%
potato, mashed, homestyle	2/3 cup	190	3	24	570	1	9.0	25.0	6	43%
potato, mashed, homestyle, w/gravy	3/4 cup	210	4	26	740	1	10.0	25.0	6	43%
potato, new, low-fat	3/4 cup	130	3	25	150	2	2.5	0.0	0	17%
potato planks, oven-roasted, low-fat	5 planks	180	3	32	370	3	5.0	0.0	1	24%
potato salad, old-fashioned	3/4 cup	340	2	30	870	2	24.0	30.0	4	63%
red beans and rice, low-fat	1 cup	260	8	45	1050	4	5.0	5.0	0	18%
rice pilaf	2/3 cup	180	5	32	600	2	5.0	0.0	1	23%
spinach, creamed	3/4 cup	260	9	11	740	2	20.0	55.0	13	69%

Food Name	Serv. Size	Total Cal.	Prot. gms	Carbs gms	Sod. mgs	Fiber gms	Fat gms	Chol. mgs	Sat.Fat gms	%Fat Cal.
squash casserole.	3/4 cup	330	7	20	1110	3	24.0	70.0	13	67%
stuffing, savory.	3/4 cup	310	6	44	1140	3	12.0	0.0	2	35%
sweet potato casserole.	3/4 cup	280	3	39	190	2	18.0	10.0	5	49%
vegetables, steamed, low-fat	2/3 cup	35	2	7	35	3	0.5	0.0	0	11%
zucchini marinana, low-fat.	3/4 cup	60	1	7	330	2	3.0	0.0	0	46%
SOUP										
chicken noodle	1 cup	130	11	12	1310	2	4.5	40.0	1	31%
chicken tortilla	1 cup	220	10	19	1410	2	11.0	35.0	4	46%
potato.	1 cup	270	8	24	1020	2	16.0	40.0	8	53%
tomato bisque	1 cup	280	4	16	1280	2	23.0	50.0	10	72%
TURKEY, breast, rotisserie, skinless,										
low-fat	5 oz	170	36	1	850	0	1.0	100.0	1	6%
BRAUM'S										
YOGURT, FROZEN										
regular	1 serving	180	3	16	35	0	3.0	0.0	0	26%
diet, sugarless, w/NutraSweet	1 serving	90	3	13	0	0	3.0	0.0	0	30%
nonfat .	1 serving	90	4	20	55	0	0.0	0.0	0	0%
'Premium Light'	1 serving	102	3	15	0	56	3.0	0.0	0	27%
BRAZIER. See DAIRY QUEEN/BRAZIER.										
BRESLER'S										
ICE CREAM, 'Royal Lites,' all flavors	1 serving	132	5	9	70	0	5.0	16.0	0	45%
SHERBET, all flavors.	1 serving	160	1	34	0	0	2.0	6.0	0	11%
YOGURT, FROZEN										
gourmet, all flavors	1 serving	116	4	22	0	0	2.0	7.0	0	15%
nonfat, all flavors.	1 serving	108	4	24	0	0	0.0	0.0	0	0%
BURGER CHEF										
BREAKFAST										
sausage biscuit.	1 serving	418	16	33	1313	0	25.0	45.0	0	53%
scrambled eggs and bacon platter	1 serving	567	21	50	1108	0	31.0	0.0	0	50%
scrambled eggs and sausage										
platter.	1 serving	668	26	50	1411	0	40.0	479.0	0	54%
'Sunrise' w/bacon	1 serving	392	19	30	978	0	21.0	384.0	0	49%
'Sunrise' w/sausage	1 sandwich	526	26	30	1412	0	33.0	419.0	0	57%
CHEESEBURGER										
regular.	1 serving	278	14	28	641	0	12.0	37.0	0	39%
double patty	1 serving	402	23	28	835	0	22.0	74.0	0	49%
DESSERT, apple turnover.	1 serving	237	2	38	0	0	9.0	0.0	0	34%
HAMBURGER										
'Big Chef'.	1 serving	556	22	37	840	0	36.0	78.0	0	58%
mushroom, single patty	1 serving	520	28	34	744	0	29.0	92.0	0	51%
regular	1 serving	235	11	27	480	0	9.0	27.0	0	35%
'Super Chef'	1 serving	604	27	35	1088	0	39.0	99.0	0	59%
'Top Chef'	1 serving	541	30	29	1007	0	33.0	100.0	0	56%
HAMBURGER MEAL, 'Funmeal'	1 serving	514	14	85	513	0	19.0	27.0	0	30%
SANDWICH										
chicken club.	1 sandwich	521	36	33	0	0	25.0	0.0	0	45%
'Fisherman's Fillet'	1 sandwich	534	26	41	0	0	32.0	0.0	0	52%

Food Name	Serv. Size	Total Cal.	Prot. gms	Carbs gms	Sod. mgs	Fiber gms	Fat gms	Chol. mgs	Sat.Fat gms	%Fat Cal.
SIDE DISH										
french fries, large.	1 serving	285	4	36	456	0	14.0	0.0	0	44%
french fries, regular.	1 serving	204	3	26	327	0	10.0	0.0	0	44%
'Hash Rounds'	1 serving	235	3	26	349	0	14.0	0.0	0	52%
salad, lettuce	1 salad	11	1	3	8	0	0.0	0.0	0	0%
BURGER KING										
BEVERAGE										
chocolate shake, medium.	1 serving	440	12	75	330	4	10.0	30.0	6	21%
chocolate shake, medium, syrup added	1 serving	570	14	105	520	3	10.0	30.0	6	16%
chocolate shake, small	1 serving	330	9	58	250	3	7.0	25.0	4	19%
chocolate shake, small, syrup added	1 serving	390	10	72	350	2	7.0	20.0	4	16%
'Coca-Cola Classic,' medium	22 fl oz	280	0	70	na	0	0.0	0.0	0	0%
coffee	12 fl oz	5	0	1	5	0	0.0	0.0	0	0%
'Diet Coke,' medium.	22 fl oz	1	0	0	na	0	0.0	0.0	0	0%
orange juice,'Tropicana'	10 fl oz	140	2	33	0	0	0.0	0.0	0	0%
milk, 2%.	8 fl oz	130	8	12	120	0	5.0	20.0	3	36%
'Sprite,' medium.	22 fl oz	260	0	66	na	0	0.0	0.0	0	0%
strawberry shake, medium, syrup added	1 medium	550	13	104	350	2	9.0	30.0	5	15%
strawberry shake, small, syrup added	1 serving	390	10	72	260	1	7.0	20.0	4	16%
vanilla shake, medium.	1 medium	430	13	73	330	2	9.0	30.0	5	19%
vanilla shake, small.	1 small	330	10	56	250	1	7.0	20.0	4	19%
BREAKFAST										
bacon.	3 pieces	40	3	0	170	na	3.0	10.0	1	69%
biscuit.	1 serving	300	6	35	830	1	15.0	0.0	3	45%
biscuit w/egg.	1 sandwich	380	11	37	1010	1	21.0	140.0	5	50%
biscuit w/sausage.	1 sandwich	490	13	36	1240	1	33.0	35.0	10	60%
biscuit w/sausage, egg and cheese.	1 sandwich	620	20	37	1650	1	43.0	185.0	14	63%
'Cini-Minis' w/vanilla icing	1 serving	110	0	20	40	na	3.0	0.0	0	25%
'Cini-Minis' w/o vanilla icing	4 rolls	440	6	51	710	1	23.0	25.0	6	48%
'Croissan'wich' w/sausage and cheese.	1 sandwich	450	13	21	940	1	35.0	45.0	12	70%
'Croissan'wich' w/sausage, egg, and cheese.	1 sandwich	530	18	23	1120	1	41.0	185.0	13	69%
French toast sticks.	5 sticks	440	7	51	490	3	23.0	2.0	5	47%
ham.	1 serving	35	6	0	770	na	1.0	15.0	0	27%
hash brown rounds, large.	1 serving	410	3	42	750	4	26.0	0.0	10	57%
hash brown rounds, small.	1 serving	240	2	25	440	2	15.0	0.0	6	56%
BUN										
hamburger.	1 serving	130	5	24	250	na	2.0	0.0	0	13%
'Whopper'.	1 serving	220	8	39	370	na	4.0	0.0	1	16%
CHEESE, American, processed	2 slices	90	6	0	420	na	8.0	25.0	5	75%
CHEESEBURGER										
bacon double	1 serving	620	41	28	1230	1	38.0	125.0	18	55%
bacon	1 serving	400	24	27	940	1	22.0	70.0	10	49%
double patty	1 serving	580	38	27	1060	1	36.0	120.0	17	55%

Food Name	Serv. Size	Total Cal.	Prot. gms	Carbs gms	Sod. mgs	Fiber gms	Fat gms	Chol. mgs	Sat.Fat gms	%Fat Cal.
'Double Whopper'	1 serving	1010	55	47	1460	3	67.0	180.0	26	60%
'Double Whopper' w/o mayo	1 serving	850	55	47	1460	3	50.0	180.0	26	52%
regular	1 serving	360	21	27	760	1	19.0	60.0	9	47%
'Whopper'	1 serving	760	35	47	1380	3	48.0	110.0	17	57%
'Whopper Jr.'	1 serving	450	22	28	770	2	28.0	65.0	10	56%
'Whopper Jr.' w/o mayo	1 serving	370	22	28	770	2	19.0	65.0	10	46%
'Whopper' w/o mayo	1 serving	600	35	47	1380	3	31.0	110.0	17	46%
CHICKEN BREAST PATTY, 'BK Broiler'	1 serving	140	21	4	570	na	4.0	90.0	1	26%
CHICKEN TENDERS										
	5 pieces	230	14	11	590	0	14.0	40.0	4	56%
	4 pieces	180	11	9	470	0	11.0	30.0	3	55%
CONDIMENTS										
barbecue sauce, 'Bull's Eye'	1/2 oz	20	0	5	140	na	0.0	0.0	0	0%
butter, whipped, 'Land O' Lakes										
Classic Blend'	1 serving	65	0	0	75	na	7.0	0.0	1	100%
catsup.	1/2 oz	15	0	4	180	na	0.0	0.0	0	0%
dip, 'A.M. Express'.	1 serving	80	0	21	20	na	0.0	0.0	0	0%
dipping sauce	1 serving	170	0	2	200	na	17.0	0.0	3	95%
dipping sauce, barbecue	1 serving	35	0	9	400	na	0.0	0.0	0	0%
dipping sauce, honey flavored	1 serving	90	0	23	10	na	0.0	0.0	0	0%
dipping sauce, honey mustard	1 serving	90	0	10	150	na	6.0	10.0	1	57%
dipping sauce, sweet and sour.	1 serving	45	0	11	50	na	0.0	0.0	0	0%
jam, grape, 'A.M. Express'.	1 serving	30	0	7	0	na	0.0	0.0	0	0%
jam, strawberry, 'A.M. Express'.	1 serving	30	0	8	0	na	0.0	0.0	0	0%
'King Sauce'.	1/2 oz	70	0	2	70	na	7.0	4.0	1	89%
mustard.	1/9 oz	0	0	0	40	na	0.0	0.0	0	0%
tartar sauce.	1.5 oz	260	0	0	330	na	29.0	20.0	4	100%
DESSERT, Dutch apple pie.	1 serving	300	3	39	230	2	15.0	0.0	3	45%
HAMBURGER										
'Big King'	1 burger	640	38	28	980	1	42.0	125.0	18	59%
'Double Whopper' w/o mayo	1 serving	760	49	47	980	3	42.0	155.0	21	50%
'Double Whopper'	1 serving	920	49	47	980	3	59.0	155.0	21	58%
regular	1 serving	320	19	27	520	1	15.0	50.0	6	42%
'Whopper'	1 serving	660	29	47	900	3	40.0	85.0	12	54%
'Whopper Jr.'	1 serving	400	19	28	530	2	24.0	55.0	8	53%
'Whopper Jr.' w/o mayo	1 serving	320	19	28	530	2	15.0	55.0	8	42%
'Whopper' w/o mayo	1 serving	510	29	47	900	3	23.0	85.0	12	41%
HAMBURGER PATTY										
regular	1 serving	170	14	0	55	na	13.0	50.0	6	68%
'Whopper'.	1 serving	250	20	0	85	na	19.0	70.0	9	68%
LETTUCE.	3/4 oz	0	0	0	0	na	0.0	0.0	0	0%
ONION.	1/2 oz	5	0	1	0	na	0.0	0.0	0	0%
PICKLE.	4 slices	0	0	0	140	na	0.0	0.0	0	0%
SANDWICH										
'Chick 'N Crisp'	1 sandwich	460	16	37	890	3	27.0	35.0	6	53%
'Chick 'N Crisp' w/o mayo.	1 sandwich	360	16	37	890	3	16.0	35.0	6	40%
chicken	1 sandwich	710	26	54	1400	2	43.0	60.0	9	55%
chicken, w/o mayo	1 sandwich	500	26	54	1400	2	20.0	60.0	9	36%
chicken, 'BK Broiler'	1 sandwich	530	29	45	1060	2	26.0	105.0	5	44%

Food Name	Serv. Size	Total Cal.	Prot. gms	Carbs gms	Sod. mgs	Fiber gms	Fat gms	Chol. mgs	Sat.Fat gms	%Fat Cal.
chicken, 'BK Broiler' w/o mayo ...... 1 sandwich		370	29	45	1060	2	9.0	105.0	5	21%
fish, 'BK Big' .... 1 sandwich		720	23	59	1180	3	43.0	80.0	9	54%
SIDE DISH										
french fries, king size, salted .... 1 serving		590	5	74	1110	5	30.0	0.0	12	46%
french fries, medium, salted .... 1 serving		400	3	50	820	4	21.0	0.0	8	47%
french fries, medium, unsalted .... 1 serving		400	3	50	760	4	21.0	0.0	8	47%
french fries, small, salted .... 1 serving		250	2	32	550	2	13.0	0.0	5	46%
french fries, small, unsalted .... 1 serving		250	2	32	480	2	13.0	0.0	5	46%
onion rings, king size, salted .... 1 serving		600	8	74	880	6	30.0	4.0	7	45%
onion rings, medium. .... 1 serving		380	5	46	550	4	19.0	2.0	4	46%
TOMATO. .... 2 slices		5	0	1	0	na	0.0	0.0	0	0%

CAPTAIN D'S
CONDIMENTS

Food Name	Serv. Size	Total Cal.	Prot. gms	Carbs gms	Sod. mgs	Fiber gms	Fat gms	Chol. mgs	Sat.Fat gms	%Fat Cal.
salad dressing, Italian, nonfat,										
low-calorie .... 2 tbsp		9	0	2	568	0	0.0	0.0	0	0%
sweet and sour sauce .... 2 tbsp		52	0	13	5	0	0.0	0.0	0	0%

ENTRÉE

Food Name	Serv. Size	Total Cal.	Prot. gms	Carbs gms	Sod. mgs	Fiber gms	Fat gms	Chol. mgs	Sat.Fat gms	%Fat Cal.
chicken, w/rice, green beans,										
breadstick, salad .... 1 serving		414	30	55	2615	0	8.0	71.0	0	17%
fish, baked, w/rice, green beans,										
breadstick, coleslaw .... 1 serving		659	36	62	1767	0	30.0	54.0	0	41%
orange roughy, w/rice, green beans,										
breadstick, salad .... 1 serving		537	35	56	2156	0	19.0	39.0	0	32%
shrimp, w/rice, green beans,										
breadstick, salad .... 1 serving		457	56	34	2194	0	10.0	191.0	0	20%

SIDE DISH

Food Name	Serv. Size	Total Cal.	Prot. gms	Carbs gms	Sod. mgs	Fiber gms	Fat gms	Chol. mgs	Sat.Fat gms	%Fat Cal.
breadstick, plain .... 1 stick		91	3	17	210	0	1.0	0.0	0	10%
green beans, seasoned .... 1 serving		46	2	5	752	0	2.0	4.0	0	39%
rice .... serving		124	3	28	9	0	0.0	0.0	0	0%
salad, dinner, no dressing .... 1 salad		27	1	3	67	0	1.0	1.0	0	36%
white bean .... 1 serving		126	8	22	99	0	1.0	2.0	0	7%

CARL'S JR.

Food Name	Serv. Size	Total Cal.	Prot. gms	Carbs gms	Sod. mgs	Fiber gms	Fat gms	Chol. mgs	Sat.Fat gms	%Fat Cal.
BACON. .... 2 strips		50	3	0	140	0	4.0	10.0	2	75%
BEVERAGE										
chocolate shake. .... 13.5 fl oz		390	9	74	280	0	7.0	30.0	5	16%
'Coca-Cola Classic' regular. .... 16 fl oz		200	0	54	25	0	0.0	0.0	0	0%
coffee. .... 12 fl oz		5	1	1	5	0	0.0	0.0	0	0%
'Diet Coke,' regular. .... 16 fl oz		0	0	0	40	0	0.0	0.0	0	0%
'Diet 7UP,' regular. .... 16 fl oz		0	0	0	80	0	0.0	0.0	0	0%
'Dr Pepper,' regular. .... 16 fl oz		200	0	52	70	0	0.0	0.0	0	0%
hot chocolate. .... 12 fl oz		110	2	22	80	1	2.0	0.0	2	16%
iced tea, regular .... 16 fl oz		5	0	0	55	0	0.0	0.0	0	0%
lemonade, 'Minute Maid' original										
style, regular .... 16 fl oz		190	0	52	95	0	0.0	0.0	0	0%
milk, 1%. .... 10 fl oz		150	14	18	180	0	3.0	15.0	2	17%
'Nestea,' raspberry, regular. .... 16 fl oz		160	0	42	40	0	0.0	0.0	0	0%
orange juice. .... 10 fl oz		140	2	33	30	0	0.0	0.0	0	0%
orange soda, 'Minute Maid' regular ...... 16 fl oz		210	0	58	20	0	0.0	0.0	0	0%
root beer, 'Barq's,' regular .... 16 fl oz		220	0	60	70	0	0.0	0.0	0	0%

Food Name	Serv. Size	Total Cal.	Prot. gms	Carbs gms	Sod. mgs	Fiber gms	Fat gms	Chol. mgs	Sat.Fat gms	%Fat Cal.
'Sprite,' regular	16 fl oz	190	0	54	65	0	0.0	0.0	0	0%
strawberry shake.	13.5 fl oz	400	9	77	240	0	7.0	30.0	5	15%
vanilla shake.	13.5 fl oz	330	11	54	250	0	8.0	35.0	5	22%
BREADSTICK.	1 stick	35	1	7	60	1	0.5	0.0	0	12%
BREAKFAST										
burrito	1 burrito	480	27	26	750	2	30.0	465.0	13	56%
cheese Danish	1 serving	400	5	49	390	1	22.0	15.0	5	48%
English muffin, w/margarine.	1 muffin	210	5	27	300	2	9.0	0.0	1	39%
French toast dips, w/o syrup	1 serving	370	6	42	430	1	20.0	0.0	3	48%
hash brown nuggets.	1 serving	330	3	32	470	3	21.0	0.0	5	57%
quesadilla	1 quesadilla	310	14	27	670	2	16.0	230.0	6	47%
scrambled egg.	1 egg	160	13	1	125	0	11.0	425.0	4	64%
'Sunrise Sandwich' no bacon										
or sausage	1 sandwich	360	14	28	700	2	21.0	225.0	5	53%
CHEESE										
American.	1 slice	60	3	0	280	0	5.0	15.0	3	79%
Swiss.	1 slice	50	4	0	250	0	3.5	10.0	3	66%
CHEESEBURGER										
double Western bacon.	1 burger	900	51	64	1770	2	49.0	155.0	21	49%
Western bacon.	1 burger	650	32	63	1430	2	30.0	80.0	12	42%
CHICKEN STARS.	1 serving	280	12	15	330	0	19.0	40.0	5	61%
CONDIMENTS. See also Salad Dressing.										
barbecue sauce.	1 pkt	50	1	11	270	0	0.0	0.0	0	0%
croutons, salad bar item	1 crouton	35	0	5	65	0	1.0	0.0	0	31%
honey sauce.	1 pkt	90	0	22	0	0	0.0	0.0	0	0%
jam, strawberry.	1 pkt	35	0	9	0	0	0.0	0.0	0	0%
jelly, grape.	1 pkt	35	0	9	0	0	0.0	0.0	0	0%
mustard sauce.	1 serving	50	0	11	210	0	0.0	0.0	0	0%
salsa	1 serving	10	0	2	160	0	0.0	0.0	0	0%
sweet and sour sauce	1 serving	50	0	12	80	0	0.0	0.0	0	0%
syrup, table	1 serving	90	0	21	0	0	0.0	0.0	0	0%
DESSERT										
chocolate cake.	1 cake	300	3	49	260	4	10.0	23.0	3	30%
chocolate chip cookie.	1 cookie	370	3	49	350	1	19.0	25.0	8	45%
strawberry swirl cheesecake	1 serving	290	6	30	230	0	17.0	55.0	9	52%
HAMBURGER										
'Famous Star'.	1 burger	580	25	49	910	2	32.0	70.0	9	49%
'Jr.'.	1 burger	330	18	34	480	1	13.0	45.0	5	36%
'Super Star'.	1 burger	790	42	50	970	2	46.0	130.0	14	53%
SALAD										
'Salad-To-Go,' charbroiled chicken.	1 salad	200	25	12	440	3	7.0	75.0	4	30%
'Salad-To-Go,' gardeb	1 salad	50	3	4	60	2	2.5	10.0	2	45%
SALAD DRESSING										
blue cheese.	1 pkt	320	2	1	370	0	35.0	25.0	6	96%
French, nonfat.	1 pkt	60	0	16	660	0	0.0	0.0	0	0%
house.	1 pkt	220	1	3	440	0	22.0	20.0	4	93%
Italian, nonfat.	1 pkt	15	0	4	770	0	0.0	0.0	0	0%
Thousand Island.	1 pkt	230	1	5	420	0	23.0	20.0	4	90%
SANDWICH										
bacon Swiss crispy chicken	1 sandwich	690	31	60	1560	4	36.0	75.0	9	47%
barbecue chicken	1 sandwich	280	25	37	830	2	3.0	60.0	1	10%
chicken club	1 sandwich	460	32	33	1110	2	22.0	90.0	7	43%

Food Name	Serv. Size	Total Cal.	Prot. gms	Carbs gms	Sod. mgs	Fiber gms	Fat gms	Chol. mgs	Sat.Fat gms	%Fat Cal.
fish, 'Carl's Catch'. . . . . 1 sandwich		510	18	50	1030	1	27.0	80.0	7	47%
ranch crispy chicken. . . . . 1 sandwich		590	24	59	1170	4	29.0	50.0	6	44%
Santa Fe chicken. . . . . 1 sandwich		510	28	32	1240	2	31.0	95.0	7	54%
SAUSAGE PATTY. . . . . 1 patty		200	8	2	480	1	19.0	30.0	17	81%
SIDE DISH										
baked potato, w/bacon and cheese. . . . 1 serving		630	20	76	1700	6	29.0	35.0	7	40%
baked potato, w/broccoli and cheese . . . 1 serving		530	11	74	950	7	21.0	15.0	5	36%
baked potato, plain. . . . . 1 serving		290	6	68	20	6	0.0	0.0	0	0%
baked potato, w/sour cream and chives. 1 serving		430	7	70	135	6	14.0	10.0	3	29%
french fries. . . . . 1 serving		290	5	37	170	3	14.0	0.0	3	43%
french fries, criss cut. . . . . 1 serving		410	5	43	950	4	24.0	0.0	5	53%
onion rings. . . . . 1 serving		430	7	53	700	3	21.0	0.0	5	44%
zucchini. . . . . 1 serving		340	5	37	860	2	19.0	0.0	5	50%

CARVEL
ICE CREAM

Food Name	Serv. Size	Total Cal.	Prot. gms	Carbs gms	Sod. mgs	Fiber gms	Fat gms	Chol. mgs	Sat.Fat gms	%Fat Cal.
'Caravella'. . . . . 1 serving		164	4	16	92	0	8.0	61.0	0	47%
'Thinny-Thin' . . . . 1 serving		92	4	16	80	0	0.0	4.0	0	0%
ICE CREAM CONE										
plain. . . . . 1 cone		25	1	5	25	0	0.0	0.0	0	0%
sugar . . . . 1 cone		45	1	10	30	0	1.0	0.0	0	17%
YOGURT, FROZEN										
'Lo-Yo' . . . . 1 serving		124	4	20	76	0	4.0	16.0	0	27%
sugarless, low-fat . . . . 1 serving		104	4	20	80	0	4.0	8.0	0	27%

CHICK-FIL-A
BEVERAGE

Food Name	Serv. Size	Total Cal.	Prot. gms	Carbs gms	Sod. mgs	Fiber gms	Fat gms	Chol. mgs	Sat.Fat gms	%Fat Cal.
'Coca-Cola Classic' small . . . . 1 serving		110	0	28	10	0	0.0	0.0	0	0%
'Diet Coke' small . . . . 1 serving		0	0	0	10	0	0.0	0.0	0	0%
iced tea, sweetened, small . . . . 1 serving		150	0	38	50	0	0.0	0.0	0	0%
iced tea, unsweetened, small . . . . 1 serving		0	0	0	50	0	0.0	0.0	0	0%
lemonade, diet, small . . . . 1 serving		5	0	2	4	0	0.0	0.0	0	0%
lemonade, small . . . . 1 serving		90	0	23	4	0	0.0	0.0	0	0%
CHICKEN PIECES										
'Chick-N-Strips' 4 per serving . . . . 1 strip		230	29	10	380	0	8.0	20.0	2	32%
nuggets, fried, 8 per serving . . . . 1 serving		290	28	12	770	0	14.0	60.0	3	44%
DESSERT										
brownie, fudge nut . . . . 1 brownie		350	10	41	650	0	16.0	30.0	3	41%
cheesecake . . . . 1 slice		300	6	23	200	0	21.0	115.0	13	62%
'Ice Dream Cone' small . . . . 1 serving		140	11	16	240	0	4.0	40.0	1	25%
lemon pie . . . . 1 slice		280	1	19	550	0	22.0	5.0	6	71%
SALAD										
chargrilled chicken garden . . . . 1 salad		190	26	12	800	4	5.0	83.0	4	23%
'Chick-N-Strips' . . . . 1 salad		370	32	21	724	4	17.0	113.0	6	42%
chicken Caesar . . . . 1 salad		230	31	5	940	2	10.0	85.0	6	38%
side . . . . 1 salad		70	5	13	0	1	0.0	0.0	0	0%
SANDWICH										
chicken . . . . 1 sandwich		290	24	29	870	1	9.0	50.0	2	28%
chicken, chargrilled . . . . 1 sandwich		280	27	36	640	1	3.0	40.0	1	10%

Food Name	Serv. Size	Total Cal.	Prot. gms	Carbs gms	Sod. mgs	Fiber gms	Fat gms	Chol. mgs	Sat.Fat gms	%Fat Cal.
chicken club	1 sandwich	390	33	38	980	2	12.0	70.0	5	28%
chicken salad	1 sandwich	320	25	42	810	1	5.0	10.0	2	14%
SIDE DISH										
carrot and raisin salad	1 cup	150	5	28	650	2	2.0	6.0	0	12%
coleslaw	1 cup	130	6	11	430	1	6.0	15.0	1	44%
french fries, potato waffle, small	1 serving	290	1	49	960	0	10.0	5.0	4	31%
SOUP, breast of chicken, hearty	1 cup	110	16	10	760	1	1.0	45.0	0	8%

CHURCH'S FRIED CHICKEN
CHICKEN

Food Name	Serv. Size	Total Cal.	Prot. gms	Carbs gms	Sod. mgs	Fiber gms	Fat gms	Chol. mgs	Sat.Fat gms	%Fat Cal.
breast, fried	4.3 oz serving	278	21	9	560	0	17.0	0.0	0	56%
breast, fried	3.5 oz	228	17	7	459	0	13.9	0.0	0	56%
breast, w/o bone	3.5 oz	252	24	5	642	0	15.6	81.9	0	54%
breast, w/o bone	2.8 oz	200	19	4	510	0	12.4	65.0	0	54%
breast fillet	1 serving	608	27	46	725	0	34.0	0.0	0	51%
breast fillet, w/cheese	1 serving	661	30	47	921	0	38.0	0.0	0	53%
leg	3.5 oz	179	16	6	348	0	10.9	0.0	0	53%
leg	2.9-oz serving	147	13	5	286	0	9.0	0.0	0	53%
leg, w/o bone	3.5 oz	247	22	4	282	0	16.1	79.4	0	58%
leg, w/o bone	2 oz	140	13	2	160	0	9.1	45.0	0	58%
thigh	4.2-oz serving	306	19	9	448	0	22.0	0.0	0	64%
thigh	3.5 oz	257	16	8	376	0	18.5	0.0	0	64%
thigh, w/o bone	3.5 oz	290	20	7	655	0	20.4	100.8	0	63%
thigh, w/o bone	2.8 oz	230	16	5	520	0	16.2	80.0	0	63%
wing, fried	4.8-oz serving	303	22	9	583	0	20.0	0.0	0	59%
wing, fried	3.5 oz	223	16	7	428	0	14.7	0.0	0	59%
wing, w/o bone	3.5 oz	284	21	9	614	0	18.3	68.3	0	58%
wing, w/o bone	3.1 oz	250	19	8	540	0	16.1	60.0	0	58%
DESSERT										
apple pie	3.1 oz	280	2	41	340	1	12.3	5.0	0	39%
frozen dessert	1 serving	180	4	27	65	0	6.0	0.0	0	30%
FISH										
fillet	1 serving	430	20	45	675	0	18.0	0.0	0	38%
fillet, w/cheese	1 serving	483	23	46	870	0	22.0	0.0	0	42%
HOT DOG										
super	1 serving	520	17	44	1365	0	27.0	0.0	0	50%
w/cheese	1 serving	330	15	21	990	0	21.0	0.0	0	57%
w/cheese, super	1 serving	580	22	45	1605	0	34.0	0.0	0	53%
w/chili	1 serving	320	13	23	985	0	20.0	0.0	0	56%
w/chili, super	1 serving	570	21	47	1595	0	32.0	0.0	0	51%
SIDE DISH										
biscuit	2.1 oz	250	2	26	640	1	16.4	5.0	0	57%
Cajun rice	3.5 oz	148	1	18	296	1	8.0	5.7	0	48%
Cajun rice	3.1 oz	130	1	16	260	1	7.0	5.0	0	48%
coleslaw	3 oz	92	4	8	230	2	5.5	0.0	0	50%
corn on the cob	5.7 oz	190	8	32	15	4	5.4	0.0	0	23%
corn on the cob, w/butter oil	1 med ear	237	4	33	20	0	9.0	0.0	0	35%
french fries	2.7 oz	210	3	29	60	2	10.5	0.0	0	43%
french fries, large	1 serving	320	3	40	185	0	16.0	0.0	0	46%
hushpuppy	2 pieces	156	3	23	110	0	6.0	0.0	0	34%

Food Name	Serv. Size	Total Cal.	Prot. gms	Carbs gms	Sod. mgs	Fiber gms	Fat gms	Chol. mgs	Sat.Fat gms	%Fat Cal.
mashed potatoes, w/gravy	3.7 oz	90	1	14	520	1	3.3	0.0	0	33%
mashed potatoes, w/gravy	3.5 oz	86	1	13	496	1	3.1	0.0	0	33%
okra	2.8 oz	210	3	19	520	4	16.1	0.0	0	62%
onion rings	1 serving	280	4	31	140	0	16.0	0.0	0	51%

COLOMBO
YOGURT, FROZEN

Food Name	Serv. Size	Total Cal.	Prot. gms	Carbs gms	Sod. mgs	Fiber gms	Fat gms	Chol. mgs	Sat.Fat gms	%Fat Cal.
French vanilla	8 oz	215	8	30	140	0	7.0	0.0	0	29%
'Gourmet'										
Bavarian chocolate chunk	3 oz	120	3	18	40	0	4.0	10.0	0	30%
caramel pecan chunk	3 oz	120	4	19	150	0	3.0	10.0	0	23%
dream	3 oz	90	3	16	45	0	2.0	10.0	0	19%
'Heath Bar Crunch'	3 oz	130	3	19	75	0	5.0	15.0	0	34%
mocha Swiss almond	3 oz	120	3	17	45	0	5.0	10.0	0	36%
peanut butter cup	3 oz	140	4	16	90	0	7.0	5.0	0	44%
'Strawberry Passion'	3 oz	100	1	18	40	0	2.0	5.0	0	19%
wild raspberry cheesecake	3 oz	100	2	18	40	0	2.0	5.0	0	18%
low-fat	4 oz	99	3	18	35	0	2.0	10.0	0	18%
nonfat	4 oz	95	4	21	70	0	0.0	0.0	0	0%
'Sundae Style'										
banana split, 'Sundae Style'	3 oz	100	2	20	50	0	1.0	5.0	0	9%
caramel fudge sundae, low-fat, 'Sundae Style'	3 oz	100	3	21	60	0	1.0	5.0	0	9%
chocolate peanut butter twist, 'Sundae Style'	3 oz	110	3	18	65	0	3.0	5.0	0	24%

COUSIN'S SUBS

Food Name	Serv. Size	Total Cal.	Prot. gms	Carbs gms	Sod. mgs	Fiber gms	Fat gms	Chol. mgs	Sat.Fat gms	%Fat Cal.
BACON	3 strips	50	3	1	145	na	4.0	8.0	2	69%
BREAD										
Italian	1 oz	85	4	12	410	0	2.0	1.0	1	22%
wheat, 2-3/4 oz per half sub	1 oz	85	5	11	450	0	2.0	1.0	1	22%
CONDIMENT, tzatziki sauce	1 serving	50	1	1	110	na	4.0	20.0	2	82%
DESSERT										
chocolate chip cookie	1 cookie	210	2	25	190	na	11.0	20.0	na	48%
cranberry walnut cookie	1 cookie	187	2	24	66	na	8.4	na	2	42%
PEPPERONI	6 slices	70	5	0	180	na	6.0	25.0	3	73%
SALAD										
chef, low-fat	1 salad	194	25	6	998	na	7.9	109.0	4	37%
garden, low-fat	1 salad	136	15	6	383	na	5.9	65.0	3	39%
Italian	1 salad	288	26	6	1063	na	17.9	106.0	7	56%
seafood, low-fat	1 salad	176	21	12	1043	na	5.9	65.0	3	29%
side, low-fat	1 salad	71	8	0	198	na	4.2	39.0	2	53%
tuna	1 salad	306	26	6	483	na	19.9	85.0	4	59%
SANDWICH										
Cold										
bacon, lettuce, and tomato sub	1/2 sub	593	20	34	1418	na	39.8	48.0	14	63%
bacon, lettuce, and tomato sub, w/o mayo	1/2 sub	337	20	34	1418	na	13.5	18.0	5	36%
cheese sub	1/2 sub	664	31	30	1636	na	46.3	87.0	23	63%
cheese sub, mini	1/2 sub	354	17	16	872	na	24.7	46.0	12	63%

Food Name	Serv. Size	Total Cal.	Prot. gms	Carbs gms	Sod. mgs	Fiber gms	Fat gms	Chol. mgs	Sat.Fat gms	%Fat Cal.
cheese sub, mini, w/o mayo	1/2 sub	228	17	16	872	na	10.7	30.0	8	42%
cheese sub, w/o mayo	1/2 sub	427	31	30	1636	na	20.1	57.0	14	42%
club sub	1/2 sub	730	50	30	2828	na	45.4	173.0	18	56%
club sub, w/o mayo	1/2 sub	494	50	30	2828	na	19.2	143.0	9	35%
'Cousins Special' sub, mini	1/2 sub	290	13	25	680	na	14.0	6.0	5	45%
ham and cheese sub	1/2 sub	622	35	30	1748	na	40.1	107.0	15	58%
ham and cheese sub, mini	1/2 sub	332	19	16	932	na	21.4	57.0	8	58%
ham and cheese sub, mini, w/o mayo	1/2 sub	206	19	16	932	na	7.4	41.0	3	32%
ham and cheese sub, w/o mayo	1/2 sub	386	35	30	1748	na	13.8	77.0	6	32%
ham sub	1/2 sub	547	29	30	1441	na	34.3	85.0	12	56%
ham sub, low-fat, mini, w/o mayo	1/2 sub	167	16	16	768	na	4.3	29.0	2	23%
ham sub, low-fat, w/o mayo	1/2 sub	311	29	30	1441	na	8.0	55.0	3	23%
ham sub, mini	1/2 sub	292	16	16	768	na	18.3	45.0	6	56%
Italian cappacolla and cheese sub	1/2 sub	567	35	30	1850	na	33.9	73.0	11	54%
Italian cappacolla and Genoa sub	1/2 sub	567	32	30	1771	na	35.5	58.0	9	56%
Italian Cousins Special sub	1/2 sub	731	43	30	2490	na	48.6	111.0	15	60%
Italian Genoa and cheese sub	1/2 sub	668	37	30	2023	na	44.5	75.0	15	60%
Italian sub, regular	1/2 sub	622	35	30	2008	na	40.0	79.0	12	58%
meatball and cheese sub, mini	1/2 sub	365	23	16	1927	na	23.1	55.0	10	57%
roast beef sub	1/2 sub	598	41	30	1571	na	34.8	54.0	12	52%
roast beef sub, w/o mayo	1/2 sub	361	41	30	1571	na	8.5	24.0	3	21%
seafood w/crab sub	1/2 sub	555	25	38	1747	na	33.6	35.0	11	54%
seafood w/crab sub, mini	1/2 sub	296	13	20	932	na	17.9	19.0	6	54%
tuna sub	1/2 sub	756	30	32	1450	na	54.3	95.0	16	66%
tuna sub, made w/o added mayo on bread	1/2 sub	500	30	32	1450	na	28.0	65.0	7	50%
tuna sub, mini	1/2 sub	495	14	22	670	na	37.0	56.0	10	70%
tuna sub, mini, made w/o added mayo on bread	1/2 sub	290	14	22	670	na	16.0	32.0	3	50%
turkey sub	1/2 sub	561	32	30	2021	na	34.8	102.0	12	56%
turkey sub, low-fat, mini, w/o mayo	1/2 sub	172	17	16	1078	na	4.4	38.0	2	23%
turkey sub, low-fat, w/o mayo	1/2 sub	325	32	30	2021	na	8.5	72.0	3	24%
turkey sub, mini	1/2 sub	299	17	16	1078	na	18.5	54.0	6	56%
veggie sub	1/2 sub	360	26	33	1590	na	14.3	35.0	7	35%
Hot										
chicken breast sub	1/2 sub	556	37	30	1391	na	31.8	33.0	11	51%
cheese steak sub	1/2 sub	470	33	46	540	na	17.0	40.0	11	33%
chicken breast sub, w/o mayo	1/2 sub	320	37	30	1391	na	5.5	3.0	2	15%
double cheese steak sub	1/2 sub	550	44	35	640	na	26.0	61.0	16	43%
gyro sub	1/2 sub	550	28	57	650	na	23.0	36.0	8	38%
Italian sausage sub	1/2 sub	816	44	30	5204	na	57.5	35.0	19	63%
meatball and cheese sub	1/2 sub	685	44	30	3613	na	43.3	104.0	18	57%
pepperoni melt sub	1/2 sub	702	41	30	1908	na	46.1	131.0	18	59%
pepperoni melt sub, w/o mayo	1/2 sub	466	41	30	1908	na	19.8	101.0	9	38%
Philly cheese steak sub	1/2 sub	510	32	43	430	na	23.0	45.0	15	41%
steak sub	1/2 sub	425	28	51	360	na	12.0	40.0	8	25%
veggie sub	1/2 sub	380	21	48	320	na	11.0	0.0	0	26%
SIDE DISH										
french fries, large	1 serving	525	7	72	464	na	24.5	21.0	11	41%
french fries, medium	1 serving	400	5	55	353	na	18.7	16.0	8	41%

Food Name	Serv. Size	Total Cal.	Prot. gms	Carbs gms	Sod. mgs	Fiber gms	Fat gms	Chol. mgs	Sat.Fat gms	%Fat Cal.
french fries, small .... 1 serving	275	4	38	243	na	12.8	11.0	6	41%
SOUP									
cheese, large .... 1 serving	330	11	23	1760	na	22.0	28.0	8	59%
cheese, regular .... 1 serving	210	7	15	1120	na	14.0	18.0	5	59%
cheese broccoli, large .... 1 serving	261	8	22	1224	na	16.5	21.0	6	55%
cheese broccoli, regular .... 1 serving	166	5	14	779	na	10.5	13.0	4	55%
chicken noodle, low-fat, large .... 1 serving	165	10	21	1444	na	4.1	28.0	1	23%
chicken noodle, low-fat, regular .... 1 serving	105	6	13	919	na	2.6	18.0	1	23%
chicken w/wild rice, large .... 1 serving	289	11	23	1691	na	16.5	28.0	3	52%
chicken w/wild rice, regular .... 1 serving	184	7	15	1076	na	10.5	18.0	2	52%
chili, large .... 1 serving	344	25	32	1485	na	13.8	62.0	6	36%
chili, low-fat, regular .... 1 serving	219	16	20	945	na	8.8	39.0	4	36%
clam chowder, low-fat, large .... 1 serving	248	12	30	1004	na	8.3	21.0	3	30%
clam chowder, low-fat, regular .... 1 serving	158	8	19	639	na	5.3	13.0	2	30%
potato, cream of, large .... 1 serving	261	7	30	1031	na	12.4	7.0	4	43%
potato, cream of, low-fat, regular ..... 1 serving	166	4	19	656	na	7.9	4.0	3	43%
red rice and beans, low-fat, large ..... 1 serving	179	7	36	1059	na	2.1	0.0	0	10%
red rice and beans, low-fat, regular .... 1 serving	114	4	23	674	na	1.3	0.0	0	10%
tomato basil, low-fat, large .... 1 serving	138	4	21	949	na	4.1	7.0	2	27%
tomato basil, low-fat, regular .... 1 serving	88	3	13	604	na	2.6	4.0	1	27%
vegetable beef, low-fat, large .... 1 serving	110	7	19	1403	na	2.1	14.0	0	15%
vegetable beef, low-fat, regular .... 1 serving	70	4	12	893	na	1.3	9.0	0	15%

DAIRY QUEEN/BRAZIER
BEVERAGE

Food Name	Serv. Size	Total Cal.	Prot. gms	Carbs gms	Sod. mgs	Fiber gms	Fat gms	Chol. mgs	Sat.Fat gms	%Fat Cal.
chocolate milkshake, large .... 1 serving	990	19	168	360	0	26.0	70.0	0	24%
chocolate milkshake, regular .... 14 fl oz	540	12	94	290	0	14.0	45.0	8	23%
malted, 'Queen' large .... 21 fl oz	889	16	157	304	0	21.0	60.0	0	21%
milkshake, 'Queen' large .... 21 fl oz	831	16	140	304	0	22.0	60.0	0	24%
vanilla malt .... 14.7 fl oz	610	13	106	230	0	14.0	45.0	8	21%
vanilla malt milkshake .... 14.7 fl oz	610	13	106	230	0	14.0	45.0	8	21%
vanilla milkshake, large .... 16.3 fl oz	600	13	101	260	0	16.0	50.0	10	24%
vanilla milkshake, regular .... 14 fl oz	520	12	88	230	0	14.0	45.0	8	24%
CHEESEBURGER									
double patty .... 3.5 oz	251	16	14	472	0	15.0	52.9	8	53%
double patty .... 8 oz	570	37	31	1070	0	34.0	120.0	18	53%
regular .... 3.5 oz	234	13	19	513	0	11.5	38.5	6	45%
regular .... 5.5 oz	365	20	30	800	0	18.0	60.0	9	45%
triple patty .... 1 serving	820	58	34	1010	0	50.0	140.0	0	55%
CHICKEN NUGGETS, all white meat .... 1 serving	276	16	13	505	0	18.0	39.0	0	58%
DESSERT									
Banana split .... 1 serving	510	8	96	180	3	12.0	30.0	8	21%
'Blizzard'									
Heath .... 14.3 oz	820	16	114	410	0	36.0	60.0	17	38%
Heath .... 10.3 oz	560	11	79	280	0	23.0	40.0	11	37%
Heath .... 3.5 oz	202	4	28	101	0	8.9	14.8	4	38%
strawberry .... 13.5 oz	740	13	92	230	0	16.0	50.0	11	26%
strawberry .... 9.4 oz	500	9	64	160	0	12.0	35.0	8	27%
strawberry .... 3.5 oz	193	3	24	60	0	4.2	13.1	3	26%
'Brownie Delight'									
hot fudge .... 10.8-oz serving	710	11	102	340	0	29.0	35.0	14	37%

Food Name	Serv. Size	Total Cal.	Prot. gms	Carbs gms	Sod. mgs	Fiber gms	Fat gms	Chol. mgs	Sat.Fat gms	%Fat Cal.
hot fudge	3.5 oz	232	4	33	111	0	9.5	11.4	5	37%
'Breeze'										
Heath	13.4 oz	680	15	113	360	0	21.0	15.0	6	27%
Heath	9.6 oz	450	11	78	230	0	12.0	10.0	3	23%
Heath	3.5 oz	179	4	30	95	0	5.5	4.0	2	27%
strawberry	12.5 oz	590	12	90	170	0	1.0	5.0	1	2%
strawberry	8.7 oz	400	9	63	115	0	1.0	5.0	1	3%
strawberry	3.5 oz	166	3	25	48	0	0.3	1.4	0	2%
'Buster Bar'										
	3.5 oz	299	7	27	146	0	19.3	10.0	6	56%
	5.3 oz	450	11	40	220	0	29.0	15.0	9	56%
'Chipper Sandwich'	1 serving	318	5	56	170	0	7.0	13.0	0	21%
'Dilly Bar'										
	3.5 oz	247	4	25	59	0	15.3	11.8	7	55%
	3 oz	210	3	21	50	0	13.0	10.0	6	55%
'Double Delight'	1 serving	490	9	69	150	0	20.0	25.0	0	37%
'DQ Frozen Cake'										
undecorated	3.5 oz	231	4	30	128	0	10.9	12.2	5	42%
undecorated	5.8 oz	380	6	50	210	0	18.0	20.0	8	42%
'DQ Sandwich'	1 serving	140	3	24	40	0	4.0	5.0	0	25%
'Fudge Nut Bar'	1 serving	406	8	40	167	0	25.0	10.0	0	54%
Ice cream cone										
chocolate	3.5 oz	162	4	25	81	0	4.9	14.1	4	27%
chocolate	5 oz	230	6	36	115	0	7.0	20.0	5	27%
chocolate	7.5 oz	350	8	54	170	0	11.0	30.0	8	29%
chocolate, chocolate dipped	1 serving	525	9	61	145	0	24.0	30.0	12	44%
chocolate, chocolate dipped	5.5 oz	330	6	40	100	0	16.0	20.0	8	44%
chocolate, 'Queen's Choice'	1 serving	326	5	40	84	0	16.0	52.0	0	44%
vanilla	3 oz	140	4	22	60	0	4.0	15.0	3	26%
vanilla	3.5 oz	162	4	25	67	0	4.9	14.1	4	27%
vanilla	5 oz	230	6	36	95	0	7.0	20.0	5	27%
vanilla	7.5 oz	340	9	53	140	0	10.0	30.0	7	27%
vanilla, 'Queen's Choice'	1 serving	322	4	40	71	0	16.0	52.0	0	45%
'Mr. Misty Float'	1 serving	390	5	74	95	0	7.0	20.0	0	17%
'Mr. Misty Freeze'	1 serving	500	9	91	140	0	12.0	30.0	0	21%
'Mr. Misty'										
large	1 serving	340	0	84	10	0	0.0	0.0	0	0%
regular	11.6 oz serving	250	0	63	10	0	0.0	0.0	0	0%
'Nutty Double Fudge'										
	3.5 oz	211	4	31	62	0	8.0	12.7	4	34%
	9.7 oz	580	10	85	170	0	22.0	35.0	10	34%
'Peanut Buster Parfait'										
	10.8 oz	710	16	94	410	0	32.0	30.0	10	40%
	3.5 oz	232	5	31	134	0	10.4	9.8	3	40%
'QC Big Scoop'										
chocolate	4.5 oz	310	5	40	100	0	14.0	35.0	10	41%
chocolate	3.5 oz	243	4	31	78	0	11.0	27.4	8	41%
vanilla	4.5 oz	300	5	39	100	0	14.0	35.0	9	42%
vanilla	3.5 oz	235	4	31	78	0	11.0	27.4	7	42%
Strawberry shortcake	1 serving	540	10	100	215	0	11.0	25.0	0	18%

Food Name	Serv. Size	Total Cal.	Prot. gms	Carbs gms	Sod. mgs	Fiber gms	Fat gms	Chol. mgs	Sat.Fat gms	%Fat Cal.
Sundae										
chocolate	6.2 oz	300	6	54	100	0	7.0	20.0	5	21%
chocolate	3.5 oz	171	3	31	57	0	4.0	11.4	3	21%
chocolate, large	1 serving	440	8	78	165	0	10.0	30.0	0	21%
strawberry, waffle cone	3.5 oz	202	5	32	127	0	6.9	11.6	3	30%
strawberry, waffle cone	6.1 oz	350	8	56	220	0	12.0	20.0	5	30%
Yogurt, frozen										
	7 oz	230	8	49	100	0	1.0	5.0	1	4%
cone, large	7.5 oz	260	9	56	115	0	1.0	5.0	1	3%
cone, regular	5 oz	180	6	38	80	0	1.0	5.0	1	5%
cup, regular	5 oz	170	6	35	70	0	1.0	5.0	1	5%
strawberry sundae	12.5 oz	200	6	43	80	0	1.0	5.0	1	4%
HAMBURGER										
double patty	3.5 oz	232	16	15	317	0	12.6	47.9	6	48%
double patty	7 oz	460	31	29	630	0	25.0	95.0	12	48%
'Homestar Ultimate'	3.5 oz	255	16	11	404	0	17.1	50.9	8	59%
'Homestar Ultimate'	9.7 oz	700	43	30	1110	0	47.0	140.0	21	59%
regular	3.5 oz	219	12	20	409	0	9.2	31.8	4	39%
regular	5 oz	310	17	29	580	0	13.0	45.0	6	39%
triple patty	1 serving	710	51	33	690	0	45.0	135.0	0	55%
HOT DOG										
'DQ Hounder' w/cheese	1 serving	533	19	22	1995	0	40.0	89.0	0	69%
'DQ Hounder' w/chili	1 serving	575	22	25	1900	0	41.0	89.0	0	66%
'DQ Hounder'	1 serving	480	16	21	1800	0	36.0	80.0	0	69%
'Super Dog' w/cheese	1 serving	580	22	45	1605	0	34.0	100.0	0	53%
'Super Dog' w/chili	1 serving	570	21	47	1595	0	32.0	100.0	0	51%
'Super Dog'	3.5 oz	297	10	21	685	0	19.1	30.2	8	58%
'Super Dog'	7 oz	590	20	41	1360	0	38.0	60.0	16	58%
SALAD										
garden, w/o dressing	10 oz	200	13	7	240	0	13.0	185.0	7	59%
side, w/o dressing	4.8 oz	25	1	4	15	0	0.0	0.0	0	0%
SALAD DRESSING										
French, diet	2 oz	90	1	11	450	0	5.0	0.0	1	48%
Thousand Island	2 oz	225	1	10	570	0	21.0	25.0	3	81%
SANDWICH										
barbecue beef	3.5 oz	176	9	27	549	0	3.1	15.7	1	16%
barbecue beef	4.5 oz	225	12	34	700	0	4.0	20.0	1	16%
chicken fillet, breaded	3.5 oz	226	13	19	400	0	10.5	29.0	2	42%
chicken fillet, breaded	6.7 oz	430	24	37	760	0	20.0	55.0	4	42%
chicken fillet, breaded, w/cheese	3.5 oz	235	13	19	480	0	12.3	34.3	3	46%
chicken fillet, breaded, w/cheese	7.2 oz	480	27	38	980	0	25.0	70.0	7	46%
chicken fillet, grilled	6.5 oz	300	25	33	800	0	8.0	50.0	2	24%
chicken fillet, grilled	3.5 oz	163	14	18	434	0	4.3	27.1	1	24%
fish fillet	3.5 oz	218	9	23	370	0	9.4	26.5	2	40%
fish fillet	6 oz	370	16	39	630	0	16.0	45.0	3	40%
fish fillet, w/cheese	3.5 oz	228	10	22	461	0	11.4	32.6	3	44%
fish fillet, w/cheese	6.5 oz	420	19	40	850	0	21.0	60.0	6	44%
SIDE DISH										
french fries	3.5 oz	300	4	40	160	0	14.0	0.0	3	42%

Food Name	Serv. Size	Total Cal.	Prot. gms	Carbs gms	Sod. mgs	Fiber gms	Fat gms	Chol. mgs	Sat.Fat gms	%Fat Cal.
french fries, large	4.5 oz	390	5	52	200	0	18.0	0.0	4	42%
onion rings	3 oz	240	4	29	135	0	12.0	0.0	3	45%

DEL TACO
BURRITO

Food Name	Serv. Size	Total Cal.	Prot. gms	Carbs gms	Sod. mgs	Fiber gms	Fat gms	Chol. mgs	Sat.Fat gms	%Fat Cal.
beef, deluxe	1 serving	440	23	43	878	0	20.0	63.0	0	41%
'Big Del'	1 serving	453	22	49	1047	0	20.0	59.0	0	39%
breakfast	1 burrito	256	9	30	409	0	11.0	90.0	0	39%
chicken	1 serving	264	13	32	771	0	10.0	36.0	0	33%
chicken, spicy	1 serving	480	23	65	1620	8	16.0	40.0	10	29%
chicken fajita, 'Deluxe'	1 serving	435	22	41	944	0	22.0	84.0	0	44%
combination	1 serving	413	21	46	1035	0	17.0	49.0	0	36%
combo	1 serving	490	26	53	1380	8	21.0	55.0	13	37%
combo, deluxe	1 serving	530	27	56	1390	9	25.0	60.0	15	40%
'Del Beef'	1 serving	590	32	45	1110	4	33.0	95.0	19	49%
'Del Beef' deluxe	1 serving	550	31	42	1090	3	30.0	90.0	17	48%
green	1 serving	229	9	32	714	0	8.0	15.0	0	31%
green, large	1 serving	330	14	46	1149	0	11.0	22.0	0	29%
red	1 serving	235	10	32	656	0	8.0	17.0	0	30%
red, large	1 serving	342	14	46	1149	0	11.0	22.0	0	29%
'The Works'	1 serving	480	18	69	1500	9	18.0	25.0	11	32%
CHEESEBURGER	1 serving	284	14	26	852	0	13.0	42.0	0	42%
CONDIMENTS										
guacamole	2 tbsp	60	1	2	130	0	6.0	0.0	0	82%
hot sauce	1 tbsp	2	0	1	38	0	0.0	0.0	0	0%
salsa	4 tbsp	14	1	3	308	0	0.0	1.0	0	0%
HAMBURGER	1 serving	231	11	26	649	0	8.0	29.0	0	33%
QUESADILLA										
cheese	1 serving	260	10	24	530	1	12.0	30.0	9	44%
chicken	1 serving	580	33	41	1240	2	31.0	104.0	21	49%
SALAD										
chicken, deluxe	1 serving	710	31	75	2130	14	32.0	65.0	13	40%
taco, deluxe	1 salad	760	31	76	2010	14	37.0	70.0	17	44%
SIDE DISH										
french fries	1 serving	242	3	32	136	0	11.0	0.0	0	41%
refried beans, w/cheese	1 serving	122	7	17	890	0	7.0	9.0	0	40%
TACO										
	1 serving	160	7	11	150	1	10.0	20.0	4	56%
beef	1 serving	210	11	11	240	1	13.0	35.0	6	57%
beef, double, deluxe	1 serving	240	11	13	250	1	16.0	40.0	8	60%
beef, double, soft, deluxe	1 serving	250	12	18	440	1	14.0	40.0	7	51%
beef, soft	1 serving	210	12	16	430	1	11.0	35.0	6	47%
chicken fajita, deluxe	1 serving	211	11	18	492	1	10.0	53.0	0	44%
chicken fajita, soft, deluxe	1 serving	210	11	16	520	1	12.0	30.0	4	50%
regular	1 serving	211	9	19	320	0	10.0	32.0	0	45%
soft	1 serving	146	5	17	223	0	6.0	16.0	0	38%
TOSTADA	1 serving	210	9	24	640	6	9.0	15.0	5	38%

DENNY'S
APPETIZER

Food Name	Serv. Size	Total Cal.	Prot. gms	Carbs gms	Sod. mgs	Fiber gms	Fat gms	Chol. mgs	Sat.Fat gms	%Fat Cal.
"Kids Heads N' Tails Cracker"	0.5 oz	70	2	9	165	0	3.0	0.0	1	38%
mozzarella sticks, 8 sticks	8 oz	710	36	49	5220	6	41.0	48.0	24	52%

Food Name	Serv. Size	Total Cal.	Prot. gms	Carbs gms	Sod. mgs	Fiber gms	Fat gms	Chol. mgs	Sat.Fat gms	%Fat Cal.
sampler	17 oz	1405	47	124	5305	4	80.0	75.0	24	51%
BEVERAGE										
apple juice	10 fl oz	125	0	33	24	0	0.0	0.0	0	0%
'Blender Blaster' Butterfinger	13 oz	768	13	97	345	0	38.0	106.0	23	44%
'Blender Blaster' kids jr.	7 oz	370	7	46	175	0	18.0	49.0	11	43%
coffee, French vanilla flavored	8 fl oz	76	0	16	4	0	1.0	2.0	1	12%
coffee, hazelnut flavored	8 fl oz	66	0	14	4	0	1.0	2.0	1	14%
coffee, Irish cream flavored	8 fl oz	73	0	16	4	0	1.0	2.0	1	12%
cola float	12 oz	280	3	47	109	0	10.0	39.0	6	31%
grapefruit juice	10 fl oz	115	1	29	0	0	0.0	0.0	0	0%
hot chocolate	8 fl oz	90	4	18	155	0	2.0	0.0	0	17%
iced tea, raspberry flavored	16 fl oz	78	0	21	0	0	0.0	0.0	0	0%
lemonade, w/ice	16 fl oz	150	0	35	38	0	0.0	0.0	0	0%
milk, chocolate, whole milk	10 fl oz	235	9	30	189	0	9.0	37.0	6	34%
milk, 2%	5 fl oz	90	5	7	70	0	5.0	19.0	3	48%
milkshake, malted, vanilla, or chocolate	12 oz	583	12	82	278	0	26.0	100.0	16	38%
milkshake, vanilla or chocolate	12 oz	560	11	76	272	0	26.0	100.0	16	40%
orange juice	10 fl oz	125	2	31	31	0	0.0	0.0	0	0%
orange-strawberry-banana juice drink, 10% juice	10 fl oz	137	0	38	0	0	0.0	0.0	0	0%
root beer float	12 oz	280	3	47	109	0	10.0	39.0	6	31%
tomato juice	10 fl oz	55	2	11	921	2	0.0	0.0	0	0%
BREAD AND ROLLS. See also French Toast.										
bagel, w/o added condiments	3 oz	235	9	46	495	0	1.0	0.0	0	4%
biscuit, w/butter	3 oz	272	5	39	790	0	11.0	0.0	4	36%
English muffin, 1 muffin, w/o added condiments	4 oz	125	5	24	198	1	1.0	0.0	0	7%
toast, dry, 1 slice	1 oz	90	3	17	166	1	1.0	0.0	0	10%
toast, herb	2 oz	170	2	15	325	1	11.0	1.0	2	59%
BREAKFAST MEAL. See also individual listings.										
'All American Slam' w/o bread, choice of potato or grits	13 oz	712	38	9	1281	1	62.0	686.0	20	75%
'Cinnamon Swirl Slam'	13 oz	1105	38	68	1374	2	78.0	635.0	26	62%
'Country Slam'	18 oz	1000	41	61	2727	1	66.0	467.0	21	59%
'Farmer's Slam'	19 oz	1200	51	82	3204	3	80.0	704.0	24	58%
'French Slam'	14 oz	1029	44	58	1428	2	71.0	777.0	20	61%
'Kids Frenchtastic Slam' w/o bread, potato, or meat	6 oz	452	19	22	664	1	33.0	311.0	9	64%
'Kids Junior Grand Slam' w/o bread, potato, or meat	5 oz	397	17	33	1118	1	25.0	230.0	7	53%
'Moons Over My Hammy' w/o bread, choice of potato or grits	12 oz	807	44	46	2247	2	48.0	430.0	8	55%
'Original Grand Slam'	10 oz	795	34	65	2237	2	50.0	460.0	14	53%
'Play It Again Slam'	15 oz	1192	51	98	3555	3	75.0	690.0	21	53%
'Sausage Lover's Slam'	17 oz	960	31	33	1934	9	68.0	480.0	22	71%
'Scram Slam'	18 oz	740	39	14	1293	3	62.0	686.0	20	72%
'Senior Belgian Waffle Slam' w/o syrup, margarine	6 oz	399	16	12	612	0	33.0	302.0	8	73%

Food Name	Serv. Size	Total Cal.	Prot. gms	Carbs gms	Sod. mgs	Fiber gms	Fat gms	Chol. mgs	Sat.Fat gms	%Fat Cal.
'Senior Triple Play' w/o bread, potato, or meat	8 oz	537	20	64	1445	2	25.0	409.0	6	40%
sirloin steak and eggs, w/o bread, choice of potato or grits	9 oz	622	43	1	632	1	49.0	572.0	18	71%
'Slim Slam' w/o topping	12 oz	495	34	98	1746	1	12.0	34.0	3	17%
'Southern Slam'	13 oz	1065	37	47	2449	0	84.0	484.0	23	69%
T-bone steak and eggs, w/o bread, choice of potato or grits	14 oz	991	73	1	1003	1	77.0	657.0	31	70%
BUFFALO CHICKEN BURGER										
burger only, w/o added condiments	13 oz	803	37	67	2143	5	45.0	77.0	9	49%
BUFFALO WINGS, 12 wings	15 oz	940	80	3	2126	2	68.0	460.0	17	65%
CEREAL, ready to eat, 'Kellogg's' average dry	1 oz	100	2	23	276	1	0.0	0.0	0	0%
CHEESE	8 oz	293	6	13	895	4	23.0	19.0	13	73%
CHEESEBURGER										
classic, burger only, w/o added condiments	13 oz	836	47	43	1595	3	53.0	137.0	19	57%
'Kids The Big Cheese' w/o fries or substitute	3 oz	334	9	28	828	2	20.0	24.0	2	55%
w/bacon, burger only, w/o added condiments	14 oz	875	53	58	1672	5	52.0	163.0	19	51%
CHICKEN DINNER										
breast, grilled, w/o salad dressing, bread	4 oz	130	24	0	560	0	4.0	67.0	1	27%
Charleston, w/o choice of side dishes	6 oz	327	25	16	993	1	18.0	65.0	4	50%
'Senior Grilled Chicken Breast Dinner' w/o bread, soup, salad, fruit, vegetable	6 oz	200	25	15	824	1	5.0	67.0	1	22%
CHICKEN NUGGETS										
'Kids Dennysaur' w/o fries or substitute	2 oz	190	9	9	340	0	13.0	30.0	4	62%
CHICKEN STRIPS DINNER										
Buffalo, 5 strips, w/o choice of side dishes	10 oz	734	48	43	1673	0	42.0	96.0	4	51%
5 strips, w/o choice of side dishes	10 oz	720	7	56	1666	0	33.0	95.0	4	54%
CHILI, with cheese topping	11 oz	401	26	21	1039	7	19.0	57.0	8	48%
CONDIMENTS										
bacon, 4 strips	1 oz	162	12	1	640	0	18.0	36.0	5	76%
bacon, peppered, 4 strips	1 oz	175	12	2	930	0	13.0	38.0	5	68%
barbecue sauce	1.5 oz	47	0	11	595	0	1.0	0.0	0	17%
cream cheese	1 oz	100	2	1	90	0	10.0	31.0	6	88%
guacamole	1.5 oz	74	1	4	264	1	6.0	0.0	2	73%
honey	0.5 oz	40	0	12	1	0	0.0	0.0	0	0%
margarine, whipped	0.5 oz	87	0	0	117	0	10.0	0.0	2	100%
marinara sauce	1.5 oz	48	1	7	206	1	2.0	0.0	1	36%
mushroom, grilled	2 oz	14	2	2	0	1	0.0	0.0	0	0%
raisins	0.75 oz	65	1	17	3	1	0.0	0.0	0	0%
salsa	1.5 oz	14	0	1	241	0	0.0	0.0	0	0%
sour cream	1.5 oz	91	1	2	23	0	9.0	19.0	6	87%
sugar, brown	1 oz	110	0	30	10	0	0.0	0.0	0	0%
syrup, blueberry flavored	1.5 oz	102	0	26	15	0	0.0	0.0	0	0%
syrup, maple favored, 3 tbsp	1.5 oz	143	0	36	26	0	0.0	0.0	0	0%
syrup, maple favored, sugar free	1.5 oz	23	0	9	71	0	0.0	0.0	0	0%

Food Name	Serv. Size	Total Cal.	Prot. gms	Carbs gms	Sod. mgs	Fiber gms	Fat gms	Chol. mgs	Sat.Fat gms	%Fat Cal.
syrup, strawberry flavored	1.5 oz	91	0	23	36	0	0.0	0.0	0	0%
tartar sauce	1.5 oz	230	0	5	185	0	24.0	17.0	3	92%
tomato, sliced, 3 slices	2 oz	13	1	3	6	1	0.0	0.0	0	0%
DESSERT										
apple pie, 1/6 pie	7 oz	470	3	64	470	1	24.0	0.0	6	45%
banana royale	10 oz	548	6	80	184	6	25.0	64.0	15	40%
banana split	19 oz	894	15	121	177	6	43.0	78.0	19	42%
'Butterfinger Hot Fudge Sundae'	9 oz	780	9	106	333	1	38.0	71.0	25	43%
cheescake, w/o topping	4 oz	470	6	48	280	0	27.0	90.0	13	53%
cherry pie, 1/6 pie	7 oz	630	3	101	550	2	25.0	0.0	6	35%
chocolate layer cake	3 oz	275	4	42	62	0	12.0	26.0	3	37%
chocolate peanut butter pie, 1/6 pie	6 oz	653	15	64	319	3	39.0	27.0	19	53%
chocolate silk pie, 1/6 pie	6 oz	650	10	60	220	2	43.0	165.0	26	58%
Dutch apple pie, 1/6 pie	7 oz	440	10	65	290	1	19.0	0.0	5	36%
hot fudge cake	7 oz	620	7	73	170	1	35.0	60.0	17	50%
key lime pie, 1/6 pie	6 oz	600	6	79	300	0	27.0	35.0	15	42%
'Kids Jr. Butterfinger Hot Fudge Sundae' ...	4 oz	341	3	46	141	0	17.0	25.0	11	44%
Oreo cookies and creme pie, 1/6 pie	6 oz	590	10	73	390	3	30.0	20.0	17	45%
rainbow sherbet	4 oz	120	1	25	30	0	1.5	5.0	1	11%
sundae, double scoop, w/o topping	6 oz	375	6	29	86	0	27.0	74.0	12	63%
sundae, single scoop, w/o topping, 'Delicious Dip'	3 oz	188	3	14	43	0	14.0	37.0	6	65%
yogurt, frozen, chocolate chocolate chip, low-fat	4 oz	110	4	19	60	1	2.0	5.0	1	16%
EGGS BENEDICT, w/o choice of potato or grits	15 oz	695	34	34	1718	1	46.0	515.0	11	60%
FISH DINNER	9 oz	732	30	48	1335	3	47.0	105.0	7	58%
'Senior Fish Dinner' w/o bread, soup, salad, fruit, vegetable	5 oz	465	15	25	743	1	34.0	68.0	5	66%
FRENCH TOAST										
plain, w/o choice of meat, fruit topping or syrup, margarine	2 pieces	507	16	54	594	3	24.0	219.0	6	44%
cinnamon swirl, w/o choice of meat, fruit topping or syrup, margarine	12 oz	1030	23	124	675	4	49.0	280.0	21	43%
GARDEN BURGER, burger only, w/o added condiments	11 oz	665	18	75	1051	8	33.0	36.0	8	44%
GRAVY										
biscuit and sausage	7 oz	398	8	45	1267	0	21.0	12.0	6	47%
brown	1 oz	13	0	2	184	0	0.0	0.0	0	0%
chicken	1 oz	14	0	2	139	0	0.5	2.0	0	36%
country	1 oz	17	0	2	93	0	1.0	0.0	0	53%
sausage	4 oz	126	3	6	477	0	10.0	12.0	2	71%
HAM, grilled, grilled slice	3 oz	94	15	2	761	0	3.0	23.0	1	28%
HAMBURGER										
'Big Texas Barbecue' burger only, w/o added condiments	14 oz	929	53	53	2271	3	58.0	163.0	24	55%
'Classic' burger only, w/o added condiments	11 oz	673	37	42	1142	3	40.0	106.0	15	53%

Food Name	Serv. Size	Total Cal.	Prot. gms	Carbs gms	Sod. mgs	Fiber gms	Fat gms	Chol. mgs	Sat.Fat gms	%Fat Cal.
'Double Decker' burger only, w/o added condiments	15 oz	1247	55	82	2200	4	80.0	125.0	13	57%
'Garlic Mushroom Swiss' burger only, w/o added condiments	15 oz	872	48	58	1529	5	51.0	116.0	14	52%
'Kid's Burgerlicious' w/cheese, w/o fries or substitute	4 oz	341	15	24	580	1	20.0	40.0	6	54%
'Kid's Burgerlicious' w/o fries or substitute	4 oz	296	13	24	368	1	17.0	28.0	6	51%
HOT DOG MEAL, 'Kids Pig in a Blanket'	5 oz	479	16	63	1684	2	21.0	32.0	7	37%
HOTCAKES										
buttermilk, w/o choice of meat, fruit topping or syrup, margarine	3 hotcakes	491	12	95	1818	3	7.0	0.0	1	13%
'Kids Smiley-Face Hotcakes' w/meat, w/o syrup, margarine	6 oz	463	14	63	1410	2	22.0	38.0	7	39%
'Kids Smiley-Face Hotcakes' w/o meat, w/o syrup, margarine	4 oz	344	7	62	1014	2	9.0	13.0	3	23%
OATMEAL										
'Quaker'	4 oz	100	5	18	175	3	2.0	0.0	0	16%
and fixings, w/o juice, bread	20 oz	535	13	115	95	7	6.0	12.0	3	10%
OMELET										
farmer's, w/o bread, choice of potato or grits	14 oz	650	29	17	1158	1	51.0	655.0	15	71%
ham and cheddar, w/o bread, choice of potato or grits	10 oz	581	37	4	1180	0	45.0	672.0	8	71%
'Senior Omelette' w/o bread, potato, or meat	9 oz	429	25	8	755	2	20.0	515.0	12	58%
'Ultimate' w/o bread, choice of potato or grits	13 oz	564	30	9	939	2	47.0	639.0	12	73%
'Veggie-Cheese' w/o bread, choice of potato or grits	12 oz	480	26	9	535	2	39.0	644.0	13	71%
PIZZA MEAL, 'Kids Pizza Party'	6 oz	400	18	47	1090	7	15.0	10.0	3	34%
POT ROAST DINNER										
w/gravy	7 oz	292	42	5	927	0	11.0	87.0	5	34%
'Senior Pot Roast Dinner' w/o bread, soup, salad, fruit, vegetable	4 oz	160	25	3	512	0	6.0	48.0	3	33%
POTATO PANCAKE, w/o meat, w/o choice of fruit topping or syrup, margarine	13 oz	530	14	59	1125	6	27.0	253.0	8	45%
SALAD										
Buffalo chicken, w/o dressing, bread	16 oz	516	33	26	1197	4	35.0	79.0	8	57%
Caesar, side, w/dressing, w/o bread	6 oz	362	11	20	913	3	26.0	23.0	7	65%
California grilled chicken, w/o dressing, bread	13 oz	277	33	10	720	4	12.0	89.0	6	39%
fried chicken, w/o dressing, bread	15 oz	438	33	26	1030	4	26.0	78.0	6	50%
garden, side, w/o dressing, bread	7 oz	113	3	16	147	3	4.0	0.0	1	32%
'Garden Chicken Delight' w/o dressing, bread	16 oz	277	30	30	785	6	5.0	67.0	1	16%
grilled chicken Caesar, w/dressing, w/o bread	13 oz	600	37	19	1792	4	41.0	101.0	10	62%
SALAD DRESSING										
blue cheese	1 oz	163	1	1	205	0	18.0	20.0	3	95%

Food Name	Serv. Size	Total Cal.	Prot. gms	Carbs gms	Sod. mgs	Fiber gms	Fat gms	Chol. mgs	Sat.Fat gms	%Fat Cal.
Caesar	1 oz	133	1	1	380	0	14.0	2.0	2	94%
French	1 oz	106	0	3	274	0	10.0	7.0	2	88%
honey mustard, nonfat	1 oz	38	0	9	121	0	0.0	0.0	0	0%
Italian, lower calorie, reduced calorie	1 oz	15	0	3	385	0	0.5	0.0	0	27%
ranch	1 oz	101	1	1	215	0	11.0	8.0	2	93%
Thousand Island	1 oz	118	0	5	170	0	11.0	15.0	2	83%
SALMON DINNER										
Alaskan salmon, grilled, w/o salad dressing, bread	6 oz	210	43	1	103	0	4.0	101.0	1	17%
SANDWICH										
bacon, lettuce and tomato, sandwich only, w/o added condiments	6 oz	634	18	37	1116	2	46.0	54.0	8	65%
Charleston chicken, sandwich only, w/o added condiments	11 oz	632	35	53	1967	4	32.0	81.0	7	45%
club, sandwich only, w/o added condiments	11 oz	718	32	62	1666	3	38.0	75.0	7	48%
grilled cheese, sandwich only	7 oz	510	19	40	1360	3	30.0	54.0	14	53%
grilled chicken, fit-fare, sandwich only	14 oz	434	35	56	1705	4	9.0	82.0	3	18%
grilled chicken, sandwich only, w/o added condiments	11 oz	520	35	64	1613	3	14.0	77.0	3	24%
ham and swiss, on rye, sandwich only, w/o added condiments	9 oz	533	23	40	1638	5	31.0	36.0	4	53%
ham and swiss, sandwich only, w/o added condiments	9 oz	497	22	34	1537	4	30.0	36.0	4	55%
Reuben, sandwich only, w/o added condiments	9 oz	580	27	37	2726	5	35.0	69.0	6	55%
'Super Bird' sandwich only, w/o added condiments	9 oz	620	35	48	1880	2	32.0	60.0	5	46%
turkey breast, on multigrain bread, sandwich only, w/o added condiments	9 oz	476	23	39	1107	5	26.0	57.0	5	49%
turkey sub, sandwich only	9 oz	476	23	39	1107	5	26.0	57.0	3	49%
SHRIMP DINNER										
'Kids Shrimpsational Basket' w/o fries or substitute	5 oz	291	10	27	774	2	16.0	68.0	3	49%
fried	8 oz	558	19	49	1114	3	32.0	135.0	6	51%
SIDE DISH										
applesauce, 'Musselman's'	3 oz	60	0	15	13	1	0.0	0.0	0	0%
banana, slices	4 oz	100	1	27	0	3	0.0	0.0	0	0%
banana, whole	4 oz	110	1	29	0	4	0.0	0.0	0	0%
baked potato, plain, w/skin	7 oz	220	5	51	16	5	0.0	0.0	0	0%
broccoli, w/butter	4 oz	65	3	7	280	3	3.0	5.0	2	40%
carrots, w/honey glaze	4 oz	80	1	12	220	3	3.0	0.0	1	34%
corn, w/butter	4 oz	120	3	19	260	5	4.0	5.0	2	29%
cottage cheese	3 oz	72	9	2	281	0	3.0	10.0	2	38%
country fried potato	6 oz	515	3	23	805	9	35.0	8.0	8	75%
french fries, chili cheese	12 oz	816	29	77	917	3	44.0	74.0	17	48%
french fries, unsalted	4 oz	323	5	44	130	0	14.0	0.0	3	39%
fries, seasoned	4 oz	261	5	35	556	0	12.0	0.0	3	40%
fries, smothered cheese	9 oz	767	27	69	875	0	48.0	78.0	17	53%

Food Name	Serv. Size	Total Cal.	Prot. gms	Carbs gms	Sod. mgs	Fiber gms	Fat gms	Chol. mgs	Sat.Fat gms	%Fat Cal.
fruit mix	3 oz	36	1	9	16	1	0.0	0.0	0	0%
grapefruit, 1/2 grapefruit	5 oz	60	1	16	0	6	0.0	0.0	0	0%
grapes	3 oz	55	1	15	0	1	1.0	0.0	0	12%
green beans, w/bacon	4 oz	60	1	6	390	3	4.0	5.0	2	56%
green peas, w/butter	4 oz	100	5	14	360	4	3.0	5.0	2	26%
grits	4 oz	80	2	18	520	0	0.0	0.0	0	0%
hash browns	4 oz	218	2	20	424	2	14.0	0.0	2	59%
hash browns, covered	6 oz	318	9	21	604	2	23.0	30.0	7	63%
hash browns, covered and smothered	8 oz	359	9	26	790	2	26.0	30.0	7	63%
hash browns, doubled, covered, smothered	13 oz	460	12	48	1213	5	26.0	30.0	7	49%
mashed potato, plain	6 oz	105	3	21	378	2	1.0	0.0	0	9%
melon, cantaloupe, 1/4 melon	3 oz	32	1	8	16	1	0.0	0.0	0	0%
melon, honeydew, 1/4 melon	3 oz	31	1	8	22	1	0.0	0.0	0	0%
onion rings	4 oz	381	5	38	1003	1	23.0	6.0	6	55%
sausage link, 1 link	3 oz	354	16	0	944	0	32.0	64.0	12	82%
sausage patty, 2 patties	3 oz	300	10	1	466	0	28.0	56.0	10	85%
strawberry-banana medley	4 oz	108	1	27	6	2	1.0	0.0	0	7%
stuffing, bread, plain	3 oz	100	3	19	405	1	1.0	0.0	0	9%
vegetable rice pilaf	3 oz	85	2	16	325	1	1.0	0.0	0	11%
SKILLET MEAL										
'Big Texas Chicken Fajita' w/o bread	17 oz	1217	49	25	1817	8	70.0	518.0	19	68%
'Meat Lover's' w/o bread	15 oz	1147	41	24	2507	7	93.0	460.0	26	76%
'Sausage Supreme' w/o bread	16 oz	1054	17	30	1740	8	83.0	430.0	23	80%
SOUP										
broccoli, cream of	8 oz	193	4	15	818	2	12.0	0.0	9	59%
chicken noodle	8 oz	60	2	8	640	0	2.0	10.0	0	31%
clam chowder	8 oz	214	5	22	903	1	11.0	5.0	9	48%
potato, cream of	8 oz	222	4	23	761	2	12.0	0.0	9	50%
split pea	8 oz	146	8	18	819	2	6.0	5.0	2	34%
vegetable beef	8 oz	79	6	11	820	2	1.0	5.0	1	12%
STEAK MEAL										
chicken-fried steak	7 oz	495	29	24	1150	1	32.0	53.0	15	58%
chicken-fried steak and eggs, w/o choice of bread, potato or grits	8 oz	430	22	9	861	4	36.0	440.0	12	72%
'Senior Chicken-Fried Steak Dinner' w/o bread, soup, salad, fruit, or vegetable	8 oz	341	16	29	943	2	18.0	27.0	8	47%
sirloin	6 oz	271	22	0	273	0	21.0	62.0	9	68%
T-bone	12 oz	642	45	1	719	0	50.0	170.0	21	71%
steak and shrimp dinner	9 oz	645	36	31	1143	2	42.0	150.0	14	59%
STIR-FRY										
grilled chicken, w/o bread	18 oz	524	34	72	1886	11	11.0	43.0	3	19%
vegetable, w/o bread	20 oz	470	13	90	1780	16	6.0	0.0	1	12%
TOPPING										
blueberry	3 oz	106	0	26	15	0	0.0	0.0	0	0%
blueberry	2 oz	71	0	17	10	0	0.0	0.0	0	0%
blueberry	cherry 3 oz	86	0	21	5	0	0.0	0.0		0%
cherry	2 oz	57	0	14	3	0	0.0	0.0	0	0%
chocolate	2 oz	317	2	27	83	0	25.0	0.0	0	66%

Food Name	Serv. Size	Total Cal.	Prot. gms	Carbs gms	Sod. mgs	Fiber gms	Fat gms	Chol. mgs	Sat.Fat gms	%Fat Cal.
fudge	2 oz	201	1	30	96	1	10.0	3.0	7	42%
nut, 1 tsp	0.3 oz	42	1	1	0	0	4.0	0.0	0	82%
strawberry	3 oz	115	1	26	12	1	1.0	0.0	0	8%
strawberry	2 oz	77	1	17	8	1	1.0	0.0	0	11%
whipped cream, 2 tbsp	0.3 oz	23	0	2	3	0	2.0	7.0	0	69%
TURKEY DINNER										
roast turkey and stuffing, w/gravy,										
w/o salad dressing, bread	14 oz	388	46	38	2467	2	3.0	116.0	1	7%
'Senior Turkey and Stuffing Dinner'										
w/o bread, soup, salad, fruit, vegetable	8 oz	220	25	25	1378	1	2.0	60.0	0	8%
WAFFLE										
'Kids Wacky Waffles' w/o syrup										
or margarine	5 oz	215	4	23	102	0	12.0	78.0	3	50%
w/o choice of meat, fruit topping										
or syrup, and margarine	1 waffle	304	7	23	200	0	21.0	146.0	3	61%
D'LITES OF AMERICA										
CHEESE, light	1 slice	53	5	2	0	0	3.0	0.0	0	49%
CHEESEBURGER										
w/bacon, on multigrain bun	1 serving	370	32	20	0	0	18.0	0.0	0	44%
w/bacon, on sesame seed bun	1 serving	370	32	20	0	0	18.0	0.0	0	44%
CONDIMENTS										
salad dressing, lower calorie	1 tbsp	40	0	1	0	0	4.0	0.0	0	90%
salad dressing, mayonnaise type										
mayonnaise, light	1 tbsp	40	0	1	0	0	4.0	0.0	0	90%
tartar sauce, light	1 tbsp	60	0	2	0	0	6.0	0.0	0	87%
DESSERT										
frozen, 'Chocolate D'Lite'	1 serving	203	6	36	0	0	4.0	0.0	0	18%
HAMBURGER										
'Double D'Lite' on multigrain bun	1 serving	450	44	19	0	0	22.0	0.0	0	44%
'Double D'Lite' on sesame seed bun	1 serving	450	44	19	0	0	22.0	0.0	0	44%
'Junior D'Lite' on multigrain bun	1 serving	200	15	19	0	0	7.0	0.0	0	32%
'Junior D'Lite' on sesame seed bun	1 serving	200	15	19	0	0	7.0	0.0	0	32%
'Quarter Pound D'Lite' on										
multigrain bun	1 serving	280	25	19	0	0	12.0	0.0	0	38%
'Quarter Pound D'Lite' on sesame										
seed bun	1 serving	280	25	19	0	0	12.0	0.0	0	38%
SANDWICH										
chicken fillet, on multigrain bun	1 sandwich	280	23	24	0	0	11.0	0.0	0	34%
chicken fillet, on sesame seed bun	1 sandwich	280	23	24	0	0	11.0	0.0	0	34%
fish fillet, on multigrain bun	1 sandwich	390	22	29	0	0	21.0	0.0	0	48%
fish fillet, on sesame bun	1 sandwich	390	22	29	0	0	21.0	0.0	0	48%
ham and cheese, on multigrain bun	1 sandwich	280	27	26	0	0	8.0	0.0	0	25%
ham and cheese, on sesame										
seed bun	1 sandwich	280	27	26	0	0	8.0	0.0	0	25%
vegetarian, 'Vegetarian D'Lite'	1 sandwich	270	16	20	0	0	14.0	0.0	0	47%
SIDE DISH										
baked potato	10-oz serving	230	6	50	0	0	1.0	0.0	0	4%
baked potato	3.5 oz	81	2	18	0	0	0.3	0.0	0	4%
baked potato, 'Mexican'	1 serving	510	27	61	0	0	18.0	0.0	0	32%

Food Name	Serv. Size	Total Cal.	Prot. gms	Carbs gms	Sod. mgs	Fiber gms	Fat gms	Chol. mgs	Sat.Fat gms	%Fat Cal.
baked potato, w/bacon and cheddar ...	1 serving	490	25	52	0	0	20.0	0.0	0	37%
baked potato, w/broccoli and cheddar	1 serving	410	15	51	0	0	16.0	0.0	0	35%
french fries, large	1 serving	320	4	42	0	0	15.0	0.0	0	42%
french fries, regular	1 serving	260	3	34	0	0	12.0	0.0	0	42%
potato skin, 'Mexi-Skins'	1 piece	99	4	6	0	0	7.0	0.0	0	61%
salad bar platter	1 salad	130	10	9	0	0	6.0	0.0	0	42%
SOUP										
broccoli, cream of	1 serving	180	8	21	0	0	7.0	0.0	0	35%
'D'Lite'	1 serving	130	14	10	0	0	4.0	0.0	0	27%

DOMINO'S

Food Name	Serv. Size	Total Cal.	Prot. gms	Carbs gms	Sod. mgs	Fiber gms	Fat gms	Chol. mgs	Sat.Fat gms	%Fat Cal.
BREADSTICK	1 piece	116	3	18	152	1	4.0	0.0	1	30%
BUFFALO WINGS										
barbecue	1 piece	50	6	2	175	0	2.0	26.0	1	36%
hot	1 piece	45	5	1	354	0	2.0	26.0	1	43%
CHEESY BREAD	1 piece	142	4	18	183	1	6.0	6.0	2	38%
PIZZA										
Deep-dish										
cheese, individual, 6-inch	1 serving	598	23	68	1341	4	28.0	36.0	10	41%
cheese, large, 14-inch diam	2 slices	677	26	80	1575	5	30.0	41.0	11	39%
cheese, medium, 12-inch diam	2 slices	482	19	56	1123	3	22.0	30.0	8	40%
ham, individual, 6-inch diam	1 serving	615	25	69	1497	4	28.0	43.0	10	40%
ham, large, 14-inch diam	2 slices	708	31	81	1868	5	31.0	53.0	11	38%
ham, medium, 12-inch diam	2 slices	505	22	57	1338	3	23.0	39.0	8	40%
pepperoni, individual, 6-inch diam	1 serving	647	25	69	1524	4	32.0	47.0	12	43%
pepperoni, large, 14-inch diam	2 slices	775	31	81	1940	5	38.0	61.0	14	43%
pepperoni, medium, 12-inch diam	2 slices	556	22	56	1397	3	28.0	45.0	11	45%
sausage, individual, 6-inch diam	1 serving	642	25	70	1478	4	31.0	45.0	11	42%
sausage, large, 14-inch diam	2 slices	787	31	83	1917	5	38.0	64.0	14	43%
sausage, medium, 12-inch diam	2 slices	559	22	58	1362	4	28.0	45.0	10	44%
vegetable, w/mushrooms, green peppers, onions, olives, individual, 6-inch diam	1 serving	616	23	70	1399	5	29.0	36.0	10	41%
vegetable, w/mushrooms, green peppers, onions, olives, large, 14-inch diam	2 slices	697	27	83	1636	5	31.0	41.0	11	39%
vegetable, w/mushrooms, green peppers, onions, olives, medium, 12-inch diam	2 slices	498	19	58	1172	4	23.0	30.0	8	40%
Hand-tossed										
cheese, medium, 12-inch diam	2 slices	375	15	55	776	3	11.0	23.0	5	26%
cheese, large, 14-inch diam	2 slices	516	21	75	1080	4	15.0	32.0	7	26%
ham, medium, 12-inch diam	2 slices	398	19	55	990	3	12.0	32.0	5	27%
ham, large, 14-inch diam	2 slices	547	26	76	1372	4	17.0	44.0	7	27%
pepperoni, medium, 12-inch diam	2 slices	448	19	55	1049	3	17.0	38.0	7	34%
pepperoni, large, 14-inch diam	2 slices	614	26	75	1444	4	24.0	52.0	10	35%
sausage, medium, 12-inch diam	2 slices	452	19	57	1015	3	17.0	39.0	7	33%
sausage, large, 14-inch diam	2 slices	626	26	78	1422	5	24.0	54.0	10	34%

Food Name	Serv. Size	Total Cal.	Prot. gms	Carbs gms	Sod. mgs	Fiber gms	Fat gms	Chol. mgs	Sat.Fat gms	%Fat Cal.
vegetable, w/mushrooms, green peppers, onions, olives, medium, 12-inch diam	2 slices	391	16	57	824	4	12.0	23.0	5	27%
vegetable, w/mushrooms, green peppers, onions, olives, large, 14-inch diam	2 slices	536	22	77	1141	5	17.0	32.0	7	28%
Thin crust										
cheese, medium, 12-inch diam	1/4 of pizza	273	12	31	835	2	12.0	23.0	5	39%
cheese, large, 14-inch diam	1/4 of pizza	382	17	43	1172	2	17.0	32.0	7	39%
ham, medium, 12-inch diam	1/4 of pizza	296	15	31	1050	2	13.0	32.0	5	39%
ham, large, 14-inch diam	1/4 of pizza	414	21	44	1464	2	18.0	44.0	7	38%
pepperoni, medium, 12-inch diam	1/4 of pizza	347	15	31	1109	2	18.0	38.0	7	47%
pepperoni, large, 14-inch diam	1/4 of pizza	481	21	44	1536	2	25.0	52.0	10	46%
sausage, medium, 12-inch diam	1/4 of pizza	350	15	33	1074	2	18.0	39.0	7	46%
sausage, large, 14-inch diam	1/4 of pizza	492	22	47	1513	3	25.0	54.0	10	45%
vegetable, w/mushrooms, green peppers, onions, olives, medium, 12-inch diam	1/4 of pizza	289	12	33	884	2	13.0	23.0	5	39%
vegetable, w/mushrooms, green peppers, onions, olives, large, 14-inch diam	1/4 of pizza	402	17	46	1232	3	18.0	32.0	7	39%
DRUTHER'S										
BISCUITS AND GRAVY	8.1-oz serving	331	6	42	1233	1	14.7	3.0	0	41%
BREAKFAST MEAL										
bacon and fried egg platter	1 serving	721	25	62	1224	2	41.9	500.0	0	52%
bacon and scrambled egg platter	1 serving	742	26	64	1243	2	43.0	501.0	0	52%
biscuit, bacon, and egg	3.1-oz serving	258	12	15	653	1	16.3	253.0	0	58%
biscuit, ham, and egg	3.5-oz serving	217	13	15	796	1	11.2	256.0	0	47%
ham and fried egg platter	1 serving	681	29	62	1622	2	35.3	511.0	0	46%
ham and scrambled egg platter	1 serving	762	27	64	1408	2	44.6	515.0	0	52%
sausage and biscuit platter, two of each	3.4-oz serving	358	12	26	894	1	22.3	34.0	0	57%
sausage and egg biscuit	3.3-oz serving	246	11	15	674	1	15.1	257.0	0	56%
sausage and fried egg platter	1 serving	741	26	63	1390	2	43.4	515.0	0	52%
sausage and scrambled egg platter	1 serving	742	26	64	1243	2	43.0	501.0	0	52%
CHEESEBURGER										
'Deluxe Quarter'	8.7 oz	660	33	46	768	1	37.6	127.0	0	52%
double patty	6.4 oz	500	29	35	618	0	26.1	105.0	0	48%
regular	4.7 oz	380	19	35	585	0	17.8	69.0	0	43%
CHICKEN										
12 pieces	3.9 lbs	5496	319	637	12904	16	171.2	902.0	0	29%
8 pieces	2.6 lbs	3664	213	425	8558	11	114.1	601.0	0	29%
breast, w/wing, dinner or snack	2 pieces	595	48	28	1607	1	30.7	154.0	0	48%
leg, w/thigh, dinner or snack	2 pieces	549	38	29	1205	1	29.8	152.0	0	50%
thigh and leg, dinner or snack	3 pieces	1281	78	90	2566	2	66.9	273.0	0	47%
thigh and wing, dinner or snack	3 pieces	1309	80	87	2465	2	70.3	271.0	0	49%
CHICKEN ENTRÉE										
breast and wing, w/potatoes and coleslaw	2 pieces	970	54	76	1899	2	49.9	159.0	0	46%

Food Name	Serv. Size	Total Cal.	Prot. gms	Carbs gms	Sod. mgs	Fiber gms	Fat gms	Chol. mgs	Sat.Fat gms	%Fat Cal.
leg and thigh, w/potatoes and coleslaw	2 pieces	925	44	77	1530	2	49.0	157.0	0	48%
FISH ENTRÉE										
	13.3-oz entrée	770	43	79	1306	4	31.3	117.0	0	37%
fried, w/fries	11.2 oz	729	42	71	1292	4	29.8	112.0	0	37%
FISH SANDWICH	4.8 oz	349	22	33	821	2	14.4	56.0	0	37%
HAMBURGER	4.4 oz	327	16	35	382	0	13.4	55.0	0	37%

DUNKIN' DONUTS
BAGEL

Food Name	Serv. Size	Total Cal.	Prot. gms	Carbs gms	Sod. mgs	Fiber gms	Fat gms	Chol. mgs	Sat.Fat gms	%Fat Cal.
blueberry	1 bagel	340	10	75	670	0	1.0	0.0	0	3%
cinnamon raisin	1 bagel	340	10	74	480	1	1.0	0.0	0	3%
egg	1 bagel	350	11	72	610	0	1.5	25.0	0	4%
everything	1 bagel	360	11	74	710	0	2.0	0.0	0	5%
garlic	1 bagel	360	11	76	720	0	1.0	0.0	0	3%
onion	1 bagel	330	10	70	660	0	1.0	0.0	0	3%
plain	1 bagel	340	10	73	710	0	1.0	0.0	0	3%
poppyseed	1 bagel	360	11	74	710	0	2.5	0.0	0	6%
pumpernickel	1 bagel	350	11	75	560	2	1.5	0.0	0	4%
salt	1 bagel	340	10	73	3030	0	1.0	0.0	0	3%
sesame	1 bagel	380	12	74	720	0	4.5	0.0	1	11%
wheat	1 bagel	330	12	73	670	4	1.5	0.0	0	4%

BEVERAGE

Food Name	Serv. Size	Total Cal.	Prot. gms	Carbs gms	Sod. mgs	Fiber gms	Fat gms	Chol. mgs	Sat.Fat gms	%Fat Cal.
'Coolatta' coffee w/cream	16 fl oz	410	3	51	65	0	22.0	75.0	14	48%
'Coolatta' coffee w/milk	16 fl oz	260	4	52	75	0	4.0	15.0	3	14%
'Coolatta' coffee w/skim milk	16 fl oz	230	4	52	80	0	0.0	0.0	0	0%
'Coolatta' coffee w/2% milk	16 fl oz	240	4	52	80	0	2.0	10.0	2	7%
'Coolatta' orange mango fruit	16 fl oz	290	0	71	30	0	0.0	0.0	0	0%
'Coolatta' pink lemonade	16 fl oz	350	0	88	30	0	0.0	0.0	0	0%
'Coolatta' raspberry lemonade	16 fl oz	280	0	68	35	0	0.0	0.0	0	0%
'Coolatta' strawberry fruit	16 fl oz	280	0	70	30	1	0.0	0.0	0	0%
'Coolatta' vanilla	16 fl oz	450	1	94	170	0	7.0	0.0	4	14%
'Dunkaccino'	20 fl oz	510	4	71	500	1	23.0	20.0	7	41%
'Dunkaccino'	18.75 fl oz	480	4	67	470	1	22.0	20.0	7	41%
'Dunkaccino'	14 fl oz	360	3	51	360	1	17.0	15.0	5	41%
'Dunkaccino'	10 fl oz	250	2	34	240	0	11.0	10.0	4	41%
hot cocoa	18.75 fl oz	440	4	75	610	3	15.0	0.0	4	30%
hot cocoa	10 fl oz	230	2	38	310	2	8.0	0.0	2	31%
hot cocoa	14 fl oz	330	3	57	460	2	11.0	0.0	3	29%
hot cocoa	20 fl oz	470	5	79	640	3	16.0	0.0	4	30%

BREAKFAST SANDWICH

Food Name	Serv. Size	Total Cal.	Prot. gms	Carbs gms	Sod. mgs	Fiber gms	Fat gms	Chol. mgs	Sat.Fat gms	%Fat Cal.
'Omwich' bagel, w/bacon and cheddar	1 sandwich	600	26	79	1630	0	21.0	295.0	8	31%
'Omwich' bagel, Spanish, cheese	1 sandwich	570	24	79	1370	0	18.0	280.0	6	28%
'Omwich' bagel, three cheese	1 sandwich	610	25	78	1630	0	22.0	305.0	9	32%
'Omwich' croissant, w/bacon and cheddar	1 sandwich	560	21	33	1190	1	38.0	295.0	13	61%
'Omwich' croissant, Spanish, cheese	1 sandwich	530	19	33	930	1	36.0	285.0	11	61%
'Omwich' croissant, three cheese	1 sandwich	560	20	33	1200	1	39.0	305.0	15	62%

Food Name	Serv. Size	Total Cal.	Prot. gms	Carbs gms	Sod. mgs	Fiber gms	Fat gms	Chol. mgs	Sat.Fat gms	%Fat Cal.
'Omwich' English muffin, w/bacon and cheddar	1 sandwich	400	21	33	1440	2	21.0	295.0	8	47%
'Omwich' English muffin, Spanish, cheese	1 sandwich	370	18	34	1180	2	18.0	280.0	6	44%
'Omwich' English muffin, three cheese	1 sandwich	400	19	33	1450	2	22.0	305.0	9	49%
'Omwich' ham, egg, cheese	1 sandwich	320	22	31	1340	2	12.0	195.0	6	34%
CINNAMON BUN	1 bun	510	8	85	420	0	15.0	10.0	4	27%
COOKIE										
chocolate chocolate chunk	1 cookie	210	3	26	110	2	11.0	35.0	7	46%
chocolate chunk	1 cookie	220	3	28	105	1	11.0	35.0	7	44%
chocolate chunk w/nuts	1 cookie	230	3	27	110	1	12.0	35.0	6	47%
chocolate-white chocolate chunk	1 cookie	230	3	28	120	1	12.0	35.0	7	47%
oatmeal raisin pecan	1 cookie	220	3	29	110	1	10.0	30.0	5	41%
peanut butter chocolate chunk w/nuts	1 cookie	240	4	24	125	2	14.0	25.0	6	53%
peanut butter w/nuts	1 cookie	240	5	24	150	1	14.0	30.0	6	52%
CREAM CHEESE										
chive	1 packet	190	3	3	220	0	19.0	55.0	13	88%
garden vegetable	1 packet	180	3	3	310	0	17.0	45.0	11	86%
lite	1 packet	130	5	3	250	0	11.0	30.0	7	76%
plain	1 packet	200	4	3	230	0	19.0	60.0	13	86%
salmon	1 packet	180	5	2	150	0	17.0	50.0	11	85%
CROISSANT										
almond	1 croissant	350	6	34	270	2	22.0	5.0	5	55%
chocolate	1 croissant	400	5	37	240	2	25.0	5.0	9	57%
plain	1 croissant	290	5	26	270	0	18.0	5.0	6	57%
DOUGHNUT										
apple crumb	1 donut	230	3	34	270	0	10.0	0.0	3	38%
apple fritter	1 donut	300	4	41	360	1	14.0	0.0	3	41%
apple n' spice	1 donut	200	3	29	270	0	8.0	0.0	2	36%
Bavarian kreme	1 donut	210	3	30	270	0	9.0	0.0	2	38%
Bismark, chocolate-iced	1 donut	340	3	50	290	0	15.0	0.0	4	39%
black raspberry	1 donut	210	3	32	280	0	8.0	0.0	2	34%
blueberry cake	1 donut	290	3	35	400	0	16.0	10.0	4	49%
blueberry crumb	1 donut	240	3	36	260	0	10.0	0.0	3	37%
Boston kreme	1 donut	240	3	36	280	0	9.0	0.0	2	34%
bow tie	1 donut	300	4	34	340	0	17.0	0.0	4	50%
butternut cake ring	1 donut	300	3	36	360	0	16.0	0.0	5	48%
cake, glazed	1 donut	270	3	33	360	0	15.0	0.0	3	48%
chcolate cake glazed	1 donut	290	3	33	370	1	16.0	0.0	4	50%
chocolate coconut cake	1 donut	300	4	31	370	1	19.0	0.0	6	55%
chocolate cruller, glazed	1 donut	280	3	35	360	1	15.0	0.0	3	47%
chocolate kreme-filled	1 donut	270	3	35	260	0	13.0	0.0	3	43%
chocolate-frosted cake	1 donut	300	3	38	370	0	16.0	0.0	3	47%
chocolate-frosted	1 donut	200	3	29	260	0	9.0	0.0	2	39%
cinnamon cake	1 donut	270	3	31	360	0	15.0	0.0	3	50%
coconut cake	1 donut	290	3	33	360	0	17.0	0.0	5	52%
coffee roll	1 donut	270	4	33	340	1	14.0	0.0	3	46%
coffee roll, chocolate-frosted	1 donut	290	4	36	340	1	15.0	0.0	3	46%

Food Name	Serv. Size	Total Cal.	Prot. gms	Carbs gms	Sod. mgs	Fiber gms	Fat gms	Chol. mgs	Sat.Fat gms	%Fat Cal.
coffee roll, maple frosted	1 donut	290	4	36	340	1	14.0	0.0	3	44%
cruller, glazed	1 donut	290	3	37	350	0	15.0	0.0	3	46%
double chocolate cake	1 donut	310	3	37	370	2	17.0	0.0	4	49%
dunkin'	1 donut	240	3	25	340	0	15.0	0.0	3	55%
éclair	1 donut	270	3	39	290	0	11.0	0.0	3	37%
fritter, glazed	1 donut	260	4	31	330	1	14.0	0.0	3	47%
glazed	1 donut	180	3	25	250	0	8.0	0.0	2	39%
jelly stick	1 donut	290	3	44	390	0	12.0	0.0	3	36%
jelly-filled	1 donut	210	3	32	280	0	8.0	0.0	2	34%
lemon	1 donut	200	3	28	270	0	9.0	0.0	2	40%
maple frosted	1 donut	210	3	30	260	0	9.0	0.0	2	38%
marble frosted	1 donut	200	3	29	260	0	9.0	0.0	2	39%
old fashioned cake	1 donut	250	3	26	360	0	15.0	0.0	3	54%
plain cruller	1 donut	240	3	25	340	0	15.0	0.0	3	55%
powdered cake	1 donut	270	3	32	350	0	15.0	0.0	3	49%
powdered cruller	1 donut	270	3	30	340	0	15.0	0.0	3	51%
strawberry	1 donut	210	3	32	260	0	8.0	0.0	2	34%
strawberry-frosted	1 donut	210	3	30	260	0	9.0	0.0	2	38%
sugar cruller	1 donut	250	3	27	340	0	15.0	0.0	3	53%
sugar raised	1 donut	170	3	22	250	0	8.0	0.0	2	42%
sugared cake	1 donut	250	3	27	350	0	15.0	0.0	3	53%
toasted coconut cake	1 donut	300	3	35	370	0	17.0	0.0	5	50%
vanilla kreme-filled	1 donut	270	3	36	250	0	13.0	0.0	3	43%
vanilla-frosted	1 donut	210	3	30	260	0	9.0	0.0	2	38%
whole wheat glazed cake	1 donut	310	4	32	380	2	19.0	0.0	4	54%
DOUGHNUT HOLE										
'Munchkin' cake butternut	3 munchkins	200	2	25	240	0	11.0	0.0	3	48%
'Munchkin' cake chocolate glazed	3 munchkins	200	2	26	250	0	10.0	0.0	2	45%
'Munchkin' cake cinnamon	4 munchkins	250	3	30	330	0	14.0	0.0	3	49%
'Munchkin' cake coconut	3 munchkins	200	2	23	240	0	12.0	0.0	4	52%
'Munchkin' cake glazed	3 munchkins	200	2	27	250	0	10.0	0.0	2	44%
'Munchkin' cake plain	4 munchkins	220	2	22	310	0	14.0	0.0	3	57%
'Munchkin' cake powdered	4 munchkins	250	2	29	310	0	14.0	0.0	3	50%
'Munchkin' cake sugared	4 munchkins	240	2	28	310	0	14.0	0.0	3	51%
'Munchkin' cake toasted coconut	3 munchkins	200	2	24	250	0	11.0	0.0	3	49%
'Munchkin' yeast glazed	5 munchkins	200	3	27	220	0	9.0	0.0	2	40%
'Munchkin' yeast jelly filled	5 munchkins	210	3	30	240	0	9.0	0.0	2	38%
'Munchkin' yeast lemon filled	4 munchkins	170	2	23	190	0	8.0	0.0	2	42%
'Munchkin' yeast sugar raised	7 munchkins	220	4	26	290	0	12.0	0.0	3	47%
MUFFIN										
apple and spice, low-fat	1 muffin	240	4	54	460	0	1.5	0.0	0	6%
apple cinnamon pecan	1 muffin	510	8	74	590	1	21.0	70.0	6	37%
apple n' spice	1 muffin	350	5	57	390	2	12.0	35.0	3	30%
banana nut	1 muffin	360	7	52	490	3	15.0	35.0	3	36%
banana, low-fat	1 muffin	250	4	57	430	0	1.5	0.0	0	5%
blueberry, 4-oz muffin	1 muffin	320	6	49	480	3	12.0	35.0	3	33%
blueberry, 6-oz muffin	1 muffin	490	8	76	610	2	17.0	75.0	6	31%
blueberry, lower fat reduced fat	1 muffin	450	8	77	590	2	12.0	65.0	9	24%

Food Name	Serv. Size	Total Cal.	Prot. gms	Carbs gms	Sod. mgs	Fiber gms	Fat gms	Chol. mgs	Sat.Fat gms	%Fat Cal.
blueberry, low-fat	1 muffin	250	4	55	430	1	1.5	0.0	0	5%
bran	1 muffin	390	11	60	620	3	12.0	20.0	2	28%
bran, low-fat	1 muffin	240	4	57	430	4	1.0	0.0	0	4%
cherry	1 muffin	340	6	53	510	2	12.0	40.0	3	31%
cherry, low-fat	1 muffin	250	4	56	430	0	1.5	0.0	0	5%
chocolate chip, 4-oz muffin	1 muffin	400	6	58	440	4	17.0	35.0	6	37%
chocolate chip, 6-oz muffin	1 muffin	590	9	88	560	3	24.0	75.0	10	36%
chocolate hazelnut chunk	1 muffin	610	10	87	610	3	26.0	70.0	8	38%
chocolate, low-fat	1 muffin	250	4	53	470	2	2.5	0.0	1	9%
corn, 4-oz muffin	1 muffin	390	8	57	590	2	15.0	55.0	3	34%
corn, 6-oz muffin	1 muffin	500	10	78	920	1	16.0	80.0	5	29%
corn, low-fat	1 muffin	240	3	52	480	0	2.5	45.0	1	9%
corn, reduced fat	1 muffin	460	10	79	900	1	11.0	75.0	7	22%
cranberry orange	1 muffin	470	8	76	600	2	15.0	75.0	5	29%
cranberry orange nut	1 muffin	350	6	52	500	3	15.0	35.0	3	37%
cranberry orange, low-fat	1 muffin	240	4	55	430	1	1.5	0.0	0	5%
honey bran raisin	1 muffin	490	7	84	880	5	16.0	30.0	4	28%
lemon poppyseed	1 muffin	360	5	56	530	1	13.0	35.0	3	32%
oat bran	1 muffin	370	11	55	620	3	13.0	20.0	2	31%

EL POLLO LOCO
BEANS
Food Name	Serv. Size	Total Cal.	Prot. gms	Carbs gms	Sod. mgs	Fiber gms	Fat gms	Chol. mgs	Sat.Fat gms	%Fat Cal.
pinto	6 oz	185	11	29	744	8	4.0	0.0	0	18%
black, smoky	5 oz	255	6	29	609	4	13.0	11.0	5	46%
black, smoky, bowl	16 oz	604	29	75	1955	6	23.0	54.0	7	33%

BEVERAGE
Food Name	Serv. Size	Total Cal.	Prot. gms	Carbs gms	Sod. mgs	Fiber gms	Fat gms	Chol. mgs	Sat.Fat gms	%Fat Cal.
smoothie, kiwi strawberry	9.5 oz	357	5	66	141	2	7.0	23.0	3	18%
smoothie, 'Minute Maid' orange	20 oz	526	9	99	198	0	4.0	44.0	7	8%
smoothie, 'Minute Maid' orange	16 oz	457	8	84	176	0	4.0	41.0	6	9%
smoothie, strawberry banana	11 oz	367	3	68	136	2	7.0	23.0	3	18%

BURRITO
Food Name	Serv. Size	Total Cal.	Prot. gms	Carbs gms	Sod. mgs	Fiber gms	Fat gms	Chol. mgs	Sat.Fat gms	%Fat Cal.
black bean, smoky	8 oz	515	15	71	1197	9	20.0	21.0	7	34%
'BRC'	7 oz	440	15	64	1105	9	14.0	15.0	5	29%
chicken, classic	11 oz	580	31	66	1595	9	22.0	108.0	7	34%
chicken, Southwest	12 oz	627	30	69	1795	5	27.0	60.0	4	38%
chicken Caesar, Mexican	11 oz	734	36	65	1214	2	35.0	79.0	8	44%
'Chicken Grande'	14 oz	648	33	72	1705	10	26.0	120.0	7	36%
'Chicken Lovers'	9 oz	476	29	47	1373	8	19.0	143.0	6	36%
'Ultimate Chicken'	12.8 oz	633	92	66	1237	5	23.0	89.0	8	25%

CHICKEN
Food Name	Serv. Size	Total Cal.	Prot. gms	Carbs gms	Sod. mgs	Fiber gms	Fat gms	Chol. mgs	Sat.Fat gms	%Fat Cal.
breast, flame-broiled, w/o bone	3 oz	160	26	0	390	0	6.0	110.0	2	34%
leg, flame-broiled, w/o bone	1.75 oz	90	11	0	150	0	5.0	75.0	2	51%
thigh, flame-broiled, w/o bone	2 oz	180	16	0	230	0	12.0	130.0	4	63%
wing, flame-broiled, w/o bone	1.5 oz	110	12	0	220	0	6.0	80.0	2	53%

CHICKEN NUGGETS, 'Dinosaur
Food Name	Serv. Size	Total Cal.	Prot. gms	Carbs gms	Sod. mgs	Fiber gms	Fat gms	Chol. mgs	Sat.Fat gms	%Fat Cal.
Chicken Bites' 4 oz	4 pieces	185	12	11	345	2	10.4	64.0	2	50%

CHURROS
Food Name	Serv. Size	Total Cal.	Prot. gms	Carbs gms	Sod. mgs	Fiber gms	Fat gms	Chol. mgs	Sat.Fat gms	%Fat Cal.
CHURROS	1.75 oz	179	3	18	221	1	11.0	5.0	3	54%

CONDIMENTS. See also Salad Dressing.
Food Name	Serv. Size	Total Cal.	Prot. gms	Carbs gms	Sod. mgs	Fiber gms	Fat gms	Chol. mgs	Sat.Fat gms	%Fat Cal.
gravy	1 oz	14	0	2	139	0	0.0	2.0	0	0%
guacamole	1.75 oz	52	0	5	280	0	3.0	0.0	0	57%

Food Name	Serv. Size	Total Cal.	Prot. gms	Carbs gms	Sod. mgs	Fiber gms	Fat gms	Chol. mgs	Sat.Fat gms	%Fat Cal.
jalapeño hot sauce, 0.5 oz	1 pkt	5	0	1	110	0	0.0	0.0	0	0%
salsa, avocado	1 oz	12	0	1	204	0	1.0	0.0	0	69%
salsa, house	1 oz	6	0	1	96	0	0.0	0.0	0	0%
salsa, pico de gallo	1 oz	11	0	2	131	0	0.5	0.0	0	43%
salsa, spicy chipotle	1 oz	7	0	1	179	0	0.0	0.0	0	0%
sour cream, light	1 oz	45	2	2	25	0	3.0	12.0	0	63%
DESSERT										
banana split	15 oz	717	12	107	310	3	28.0	56.0	11	35%
cheesecake	3.5 oz	310	8	30	228	0	18.0	58.0	9	52%
'Foster's Freeze' w/o topping	4.6 oz	180	4	30	100	0	5.0	20.0	3	25%
SALAD										
'Pollo Bowl'	17 oz	469	30	66	1868	8	11.0	42.0	2	21%
bowl, flame-broiled chicken	12 oz	357	25	39	1079	4	13.0	42.0	2	31%
bowl, Mexican Caesar chicken	11 oz	491	25	32	1170	2	30.0	55.0	6	54%
bowl, Southwest chicken	13 oz	529	25	40	1332	4	31.0	52.0	5	52%
garden, large	14 oz	225	14	17	214	4	13.0	30.0	6	49%
garden, regular	4 oz	105	5	7	99	1	7.0	15.0	3	57%
tostada, w/o shell and sour cream	14 oz	304	29	28	1175	4	11.0	57.0	3	30%
SALAD DRESSING										
blue cheese	2 oz	300	2	2	590	0	32.0	50.0	6	95%
cilantro, creamy	1.75 oz	266	1	1	306	0	29.0	13.0	4	97%
Italian, light	2 oz	25	0	3	990	0	1.0	0.0	1	43%
ranch	2 oz	350	1	2	500	0	39.0	5.0	6	97%
Southwest	1.75 oz	301	0	2	443	0	32.0	18.0	4	97%
Thousand Island	2 oz	270	1	9	460	0	27.0	30.0	4	86%
SIDE DISH. See also Beans.										
coleslaw	5 oz	206	2	12	358	2	16.0	11.0	3	72%
corn cobbette	3 oz	80	3	18	10	1	1.0	0.0	0	10%
french fries	5.5 oz	444	6	61	605	0	19.0	0.0	5	39%
macaroni and cheese	1 serving	330	14	32	1290	4	16.0	30.0	6	44%
mashed potato	5 oz	97	3	21	369	2	1.0	0.0	0	9%
potato salad	6 oz	256	3	30	527	3	14.0	15.0	2	49%
Spanish rice	4 oz	130	2	24	397	1	3.0	0.0	1	21%
vegetables, fresh	4 oz	57	2	8	79	3	2.0	0.0	1	31%
TACO										
'Al Carbon'	3 oz	164	13	14	21	1	6.0	68.0	2	33%
chicken, soft	4.5 oz	237	17	15	629	0	12.0	74.0	4	46%
taquito, chicken	5 oz	370	15	43	690	3	17.0	25.0	4	40%
TORTILLA										
corn, 6-inch diam	1 oz	70	1	14	35	1	1.0	0.0	0	13%
corn, 4.5-inch diam	0.5 oz	32	1	6	21	0	0.5	0.0	0	14%
flour, 11-inch diam	3 oz	260	7	42	583	6	7.0	0.0	2	24%
flour, 6-inch diam	1 oz	90	3	13	224	0	3.0	0.0	0	30%
spicy tomato	3 oz	254	7	42	577	2	6.0	0.0	1	22%
TORTILLA CHIPS, no salt	5 oz	760	9	86	22	7	42.0	0.0	10	50%
TOSTADA SHELL	5.6 oz	440	7	42	610	0	27.0	0.0	4	55%
EVERYTHING YOGURT										
YOGURT, FROZEN										
low-fat	1 serving	95	3	18	30	0	1.0	5.0	0	10%
nonfat	1 serving	80	3	17	40	0	0.0	0.0	0	0%

Food Name	Serv. Size	Total Cal.	Prot. gms	Carbs gms	Sod. mgs	Fiber gms	Fat gms	Chol. mgs	Sat.Fat gms	%Fat Cal.
GODFATHER'S PIZZA										
PIZZA										
Cheese										
golden crust, large	1/10 pizza	261	8	31	314	0	11.0	23.0	0	39%
golden crust, medium	1/8 pizza	229	8	28	272	0	9.0	19.0	0	36%
golden crust, small	1/6 pizza	213	8	27	258	0	8.0	19.0	0	34%
original crust, large	1/10 pizza	271	12	37	329	0	8.0	28.0	0	27%
original crust, medium	1/8 pizza	242	10	35	285	0	7.0	22.0	0	26%
original crust, mini	1/4 pizza	138	6	20	159	0	4.0	13.0	0	26%
original crust, small	1/6 pizza	239	10	32	289	0	7.0	25.0	0	27%
thin crust, large	1/10 pizza	228	11	28	464	0	7.0	16.0	0	29%
thin crust, medium	1/8 pizza	210	10	26	410	0	7.0	14.0	0	30%
thin crust, small	1/6 pizza	180	9	21	370	0	6.0	10.0	0	31%
Combo										
golden crust, large	1/10 pizza	322	14	33	602	0	15.0	34.0	0	42%
golden crust, medium	1/8 pizza	283	13	30	526	0	13.0	29.0	0	40%
golden crust, small	1/6 pizza	273	13	29	542	0	12.0	31.0	0	39%
original crust, large	1/10 pizza	332	16	39	617	0	12.0	39.0	0	33%
original crust, medium	1/8 pizza	318	16	37	569	0	12.0	38.0	0	34%
original crust, mini	1/4 pizza	164	8	21	287	0	5.0	17.0	0	28%
original crust, small	1/6 pizza	299	15	34	573	0	11.0	37.0	0	34%
thin crust, large	1/10 pizza	336	17	31	870	0	16.0	27.0	0	43%
thin crust, medium	1/8 pizza	310	15	29	790	0	14.0	25.0	0	42%
thin crust, small	1/6 pizza	270	13	23	710	0	13.0	25.0	0	45%
STUFFED PIZZA										
cheese, large	1/10 pizza	381	16	44	677	0	16.0	32.0	0	38%
cheese, medium	1/8 pizza	350	14	42	610	0	13.0	25.0	0	34%
cheese, small	1/6 pizza	310	13	38	560	0	11.0	25.0	0	33%
combo, large	1/10 pizza	521	23	47	1204	0	26.0	48.0	0	46%
combo, medium	1/8 pizza	480	21	45	1105	0	23.0	43.0	0	44%
combo, small	1/6 pizza	430	19	41	1000	0	20.0	40.0	0	43%
GOLDEN CORRAL										
BREAD, 'Texas Toast'	1 serving	170	5	26	230	0	6.0	0.0	0	30%
CHICKEN										
fillet, 'Golden Fried'	1 serving	370	37	14	570	0	19.0	85.0	0	46%
fillet, 'Golden Grilled'	1 serving	170	32	0	520	0	5.0	100.0	0	26%
POTATO, baked	1 serving	220	5	46	60	0	2.0	0.0	0	8%
RIBEYE STEAK, regular	1 serving	450	34	0	220	0	35.0	120.0	0	70%
SHRIMP, 'Golden Fried'	1 serving	250	12	24	470	0	12.0	90.0	0	43%
SIRLOIN STEAK										
	5-oz serving	230	27	0	270	0	14.0	85.0	0	54%
chopped	4-oz serving	320	28	0	160	0	23.0	100.0	0	65%
tips, w/onions and pepper	8.2-oz serving	290	30	8	260	0	13.0	120.0	0	43%
HARDEE'S										
BEVERAGE										
chocolate shake	12.3 fl oz	370	13	67	270	na	5.0	30.0	3	12%
orange juice	10 fl oz	140	2	34	5	na	0.0	0.0	0	0%
vanilla shake	12.3 fl oz	350	12	65	300	na	5.0	20.0	3	13%

Food Name	Serv. Size	Total Cal.	Prot. gms	Carbs gms	Sod. mgs	Fiber gms	Fat gms	Chol. mgs	Sat.Fat gms	%Fat Cal.
BISCUIT										
and gravy	1 serving	530	10	56	1550	na	30.0	15.0	9	51%
apple cinnamon n' raisin	1 serving	250	2	42	350	na	8.0	0.0	2	29%
jelly	1 serving	440	6	57	1000	na	21.0	0.0	6	43%
chicken	1 sandwich	590	24	62	1820	na	27.0	45.0	7	41%
country ham	1 sandwich	440	14	44	1710	na	22.0	30.0	7	46%
egg and cheese	1 sandwich	520	17	45	1420	na	30.0	210.0	11	52%
ham	1 sandwich	410	13	45	1200	na	20.0	25.0	6	44%
'Made From Scratch'	1 serving	390	6	44	1000	na	21.0	0.0	6	49%
omelet	1 sandwich	550	20	45	1350	na	32.0	225.0	12	53%
plain or buttermilk	1 biscuit	353	6	47	1020	1	16.0	2.4	1	40%
sausage and egg	1 sandwich	620	19	45	1370	na	41.0	225.0	13	59%
sausage biscuit	1 sandwich	550	12	44	1310	na	36.0	25.0	11	59%
steak	1 sandwich	580	15	56	1580	na	32.0	30.0	10	50%
CHICKEN										
breast, w/o bone	1 serving	370	29	29	1190	na	15.0	75.0	4	37%
leg, w/o bone	1 serving	170	13	15	570	na	7.0	45.0	2	36%
thigh, w/o bone	1 serving	330	19	30	1000	na	15.0	60.0	4	41%
wing, w/o bone	1 serving	200	10	23	740	na	8.0	30.0	2	35%
DESSERT										
apple turnover	1 serving	270	4	38	250	na	12.0	0.0	4	39%
cone, twist	1 serving	180	4	34	120	na	2.0	10.0	1	11%
peach cobbler	1 serving	310	2	60	360	na	7.0	0.0	1	20%
GRAVY	1 serving	20	0	3	260	na	0.0	0.0	0	0%
HAMBURGER										
'All-Star'	1 burger	660	29	41	1260	na	43.0	100.0	14	58%
'Famous Star'	1 burger	570	24	41	860	na	35.0	80.0	10	55%
'Frisco Burger'	1 burger	720	31	37	1180	na	49.0	95.0	15	62%
'Monster Burger'	1 burger	1060	49	37	1860	na	79.0	185.0	29	67%
regular	1 burger	270	13	29	550	na	11.0	35.0	4	37%
'Super Star'	1 burger	790	40	41	970	na	53.0	145.0	17	60%
HOT DOG, w/condiments	1 serving	450	15	25	1240	na	32.0	55.0	12	64%
SANDWICH										
bacon Swiss crispy chicken	1 sandwich	670	24	45	1600	na	44.0	55.0	9	59%
chicken fillet	1 sandwich	480	24	44	1190	na	23.0	55.0	4	43%
chicken, grilled	1 sandwich	350	23	28	860	na	16.0	65.0	3	41%
'Fisherman's Fillet'	1 sandwich	530	25	45	1280	na	28.0	75.0	7	47%
'Frisco Ham'	1 sandwich	450	22	42	1290	na	22.0	225.0	8	44%
ham and cheese, hot	1 sandwich	300	16	34	1390	na	12.0	50.0	6	35%
roast beef, big	1 sandwich	410	24	26	1140	na	24.0	40.0	9	52%
roast beef, monster	1 sandwich	610	35	26	1940	na	39.0	105.0	18	59%
roast beef, regular	1 sandwich	310	17	26	800	na	16.0	40.0	6	46%
SIDE DISH										
coleslaw	1 serving	240	2	13	340	na	20.0	10.0	3	75%
crispy curl potatoes, large	1 serving	520	7	62	1450	na	28.0	0.0	5	48%
crispy curl potatoes, medium	1 serving	340	5	41	950	na	18.0	0.0	4	47%
crispy curl potatoes, monster	1 serving	590	8	70	1640	na	31.0	0.0	6	47%
french fries, large	1 serving	440	5	59	520	na	21.0	0.0	3	42%
french fries, monster	1 serving	510	6	67	590	na	24.0	0.0	3	43%
french fries, regular	1 serving	340	4	45	390	na	16.0	0.0	2	42%

Food Name	Serv. Size	Total Cal.	Prot. gms	Carbs gms	Sod. mgs	Fiber gms	Fat gms	Chol. mgs	Sat.Fat gms	%Fat Cal.
hash rounds, regular	1 serving	230	3	24	560	na	14.0	0.0	3	54%
mashed potato, small	1 serving	70	2	14	330	na	0.0	0.0	0	0%

HARVEY'S FOODS

BREAKFAST

pancake	1 serving	89	2	17	0	0	1.0	8.0	0	11%
sausage	1 serving	167	9	3	0	0	14.0	12.0	0	72%
toast, plain	1 serving	250	8	48	0	0	3.0	0.0	0	11%
CHEESEBURGER	1 serving	415	22	41	0	0	18.0	30.0	0	39%
CHICKEN FINGERS	1 serving	240	15	18	0	0	12.0	57.0	0	45%
DESSERT, apple turnover	1 serving	179	1	28	0	0	7.0	7.0	0	35%

HAMBURGER

double	1 burger	530	31	44	0	0	26.0	34.0	0	44%
regular	1 burger	355	18	40	0	0	14.0	17.0	0	35%
super	1 burger	477	37	38	0	0	19.0	112.0	0	36%
HOT DOG	1 serving	332	12	32	0	0	15.0	50.0	0	43%

MUFFIN

blueberry	1 muffin	254	4	45	0	0	6.0	0.0	0	22%
bran	1 muffin	301	5	42	0	0	13.0	0.0	0	38%

SANDWICH

chicken	1 sandwich	419	19	46	0	0	16.0	110.0	0	36%
'Western'	1 sandwich	347	15	58	0	0	10.0	265.0	0	24%

SIDE DISH

french fries	1 serving	478	10	56	0	0	24.0	5.0	0	45%
hash browns	1 serving	146	2	15	0	0	9.0	2.0	0	54%
onion rings	1 serving	288	4	36	0	0	14.0	5.0	0	44%

HUNGRY HUNTER

CHICKEN, breast, teriyaki, boneless, charbroiled	1 serving	413	71	9	237	0	8.0	193.0	0	18%

CRAB

Alaskan king, w/1 tbsp butter	1 serving	432	73	0	3436	0	13.0	194.0	0	29%
Alaskan king, w/o butter	1 serving	332	73	0	3319	0	2.0	163.0	0	6%

LOBSTER

cooked, w/o butter	1 serving	139	29	2	539	0	1.0	102.0	0	7%
cooked, w/1 tbsp. butter	1 serving	241	29	2	657	0	12.0	133.0	0	47%

SIDE DISH

baked potato	1 serving	185	4	43	13	4	0.0	0.0	0	0%
rice pilaf	1 serving	142	4	26	223	1	2.0	0.0	0	13%
SNAPPER, RED, fresh, cooked in 1/2 oz. butter	1 serving	329	47	0	262	0	15.0	114.0	0	42%

STEAK

filet mignon	8 oz	539	69	0	150	0	27.0	203.0	0	47%
filet mignon, choice	3.5 oz	238	30	0	66	0	11.9	89.5	0	47%

IN-N-OUT

BEVERAGE

chocolate shake	15 fl oz	690	9	83	350	0	36.0	95.0	24	47%
'Coca-Cola Classic'	16 fl oz	198	0	54	12	0	0.0	0.0	0	0%
coffee	10 fl oz	5	0	1	3	0	0.0	0.0	0	0%

Food Name	Serv. Size	Total Cal.	Prot. gms	Carbs gms	Sod. mgs	Fiber gms	Fat gms	Chol. mgs	Sat.Fat gms	%Fat Cal.
'Diet Coke'	16 fl oz	0	0	0	20	0	0.0	0.0	0	0%
'Dr Pepper'	16 fl oz	200	0	52	0	0	0.0	0.0	0	0%
iced tea	16 fl oz	0	0	0	0	0	0.0	0.0	0	0%
lemonade	16 fl oz	180	0	40	20	0	0.0	0.0	0	0%
milk	10 fl oz	180	12	18	190	0	6.0	30.0	4	31%
root beer	16 fl oz	222	0	60	48	0	0.0	0.0	0	0%
'7UP'	16 fl oz	220	0	52	40	0	0.0	0.0	0	0%
strawberry shake	15 fl oz	690	8	91	280	2	33.0	85.0	22	43%
vanilla shake	15 fl oz	680	9	78	390	2	37.0	90.0	25	49%
CHEESEBURGER										
'Protein Style' w/lettuce leaves, w/o bun	1 serving	330	18	11	720	2	25.0	60.0	9	66%
regular	1 serving	480	22	39	1000	3	27.0	60.0	10	50%
w/o spread, w/mustard and ketchup	1 serving	400	22	41	1080	3	18.0	55.0	9	39%
HAMBURGER										
'Double Double'	1 serving	670	37	40	1430	3	41.0	120.0	18	55%
'Double Double' protein style, w/lettuce leaves, w/o bun	1 serving	520	33	11	1160	2	39.0	120.0	17	67%
'Double Double' w/o spread, w/mustard and ketchup	1 serving	590	37	42	1510	3	32.0	115.0	17	48%
regular	1 serving	390	16	39	640	3	19.0	40.0	5	44%
regular, protein style, w/lettuce leaves, w/o bun	1 serving	240	12	10	370	2	17.0	40.0	5	63%
regular, w/o spread, w/mustard and ketchup	1 serving	310	16	41	720	3	10.0	35.0	4	28%
SIDE DISH, french fries	1 serving	400	7	54	245	2	18.0	0.0	5	40%

JACK IN THE BOX

BEVERAGE

Food Name	Serv. Size	Total Cal.	Prot. gms	Carbs gms	Sod. mgs	Fiber gms	Fat gms	Chol. mgs	Sat.Fat gms	%Fat Cal.
cappuccino ice cream shake, regular	16 fl oz	630	11	80	320	0	29.0	90.0	17	42%
chocolate ice cream shake, regular	16 fl oz	630	11	85	330	0	27.0	85.0	16	39%
'Coca-Cola Classic' regular	20 fl oz	170	0	46	8	0	0.0	0.0	0	0%
coffee, regular	12 fl oz	5	0	1	5	0	0.0	0.0	0	0%
'Diet Coke' regular	20 fl oz	0	0	0	15	0	0.0	0.0	0	0%
'Dr Pepper' regular	20 fl oz	190	0	49	25	0	0.0	0.0	0	0%
iced tea, regular	20 fl oz	0	0	0	0	0	0.0	0.0	0	0%
lemonade, 'Minute Maid' regular	20 fl oz	190	0	65	100	0	0.0	0.0	0	0%
milk, 2%	8 fl oz	130	9	14	85	0	5.0	25.0	3	33%
orange juice	10 fl oz	150	2	34	20	1	0.0	0.0	0	0%
Oreo cookie ice cream shake, regular	16 fl oz	740	13	91	490	2	36.0	95.0	19	44%
root beer, 'Barq's' regular	20 fl oz	180	0	50	40	0	0.0	0.0	0	0%
'Sprite' regular	20 fl oz	160	0	41	40	0	0.0	0.0	0	0%
BREAKFAST										
'Breakfast Jack'	1 sandwich	280	17	28	750	1	12.0	190.0	5	38%
French toast sticks, w/bacon	1 serving	470	12	53	700	2	23.0	30.0	4	44%
pancake, w/bacon	1 serving	370	12	59	1020	3	9.0	30.0	2	22%
sausage croissant	1 serving	700	21	38	1000	0	51.0	240.0	20	66%
'Supreme Croissant'	1 sandwich	530	22	37	960	0	32.0	225.0	13	55%
'Ultimate Breakfast Sandwich'	1 sandwich	600	34	39	1470	2	34.0	400.0	10	51%
CHEESE										
American	1 slice	45	2	1	230	0	4.0	10.0	2	75%

Food Name	Serv. Size	Total Cal.	Prot. gms	Carbs gms	Sod. mgs	Fiber gms	Fat gms	Chol. mgs	Sat.Fat gms	%Fat Cal.
Swiss style	1 slice	40	2	1	210	0	4.0	10.0	2	75%
CHEESEBURGER										
'Bacon Ultimate'	1 burger	1020	58	37	1740	1	71.0	210.0	26	63%
double patty	1 burger	460	24	32	1090	2	27.0	80.0	12	52%
'Jumbo Jack'	1 burger	680	31	39	1130	2	45.0	115.0	16	59%
regular	1 burger	320	14	30	720	2	16.0	40.0	6	45%
'Ultimate'	1 burger	950	52	37	1370	1	66.0	195.0	26	63%
CHICKEN, breast pieces	5 pieces	360	27	24	970	1	17.0	80.0	3	43%
CHICKEN MEAL										
chicken teriyaki bowl	1 serving	670	26	128	1730	3	4.0	15.0	1	6%
4 chicken pieces, w/french fries	1 serving	730	26	79	1690	5	34.0	65.0	7	42%
CONDIMENTS. See also Salad Dressing.										
barbecue dipping sauce	1 serving	45	1	11	310	0	0.0	0.0	0	0%
buttermilk dipping house sauce	1 serving	130	1	3	240	1	13.0	10.0	5	88%
catsup	1 serving	10	0	2	105	0	0.0	0.0	0	0%
croutons, salad bar item	1 serving	50	1	8	105	0	2.0	0.0	1	33%
jelly, grape	1 serving	40	0	10	5	0	0.0	0.0	0	0%
margarine-like spread, 'Country Crock'	1 serving	25	0	0	45	0	2.5	0.0	1	100%
salsa	1 serving	10	0	2	200	0	0.0	0.0	0	0%
sour cream	1 serving	60	1	1	30	0	6.0	20.0	4	87%
soy sauce	1 serving	5	1	1	480	0	0.0	0.0	0	0%
sweet and sour sauce	1 serving	45	1	11	160	0	0.0	0.0	0	0%
syrup	1 serving	130	0	30	5	0	0.0	0.0	0	0%
tartar sauce	1 serving	210	1	2	340	0	22.0	30.0	3	94%
DESSERT										
apple turnover, hot	1 serving	340	4	41	510	2	18.0	0.0	4	47%
carrot cake	1 serving	370	3	54	340	2	16.0	40.0	3	39%
double fudge cake	1 serving	300	3	50	320	1	10.0	50.0	2	30%
cheesecake	1 serving	320	7	32	220	1	18.0	65.0	10	51%
strawberry ice cream, regular	16 fl oz	640	10	85	300	0	28.0	85.0	15	40%
vanilla ice cream, regular	16 fl oz	610	12	73	320	0	31.0	95.0	18	45%
FISH AND CHIPS	1 serving	780	19	86	1740	6	39.0	45.0	9	46%
HAMBURGER										
'Jumbo Jack'	1 burger	590	27	39	670	2	37.0	90.0	11	56%
regular	1 burger	280	12	30	490	2	12.0	30.0	4	39%
'Sourdough Jack'	1 burger	690	34	37	1180	2	45.0	105.0	15	59%
SALAD										
chicken garden	1 salad	200	23	8	420	3	9.0	65.0	4	40%
side	1 salad	50	2	3	75	1	3.0	10.0	2	57%
SALAD DRESSING										
blue cheese	1 serving	210	1	11	750	0	15.0	25.0	3	74%
house, buttermilk	1 serving	290	1	6	560	0	30.0	20.0	11	91%
Italian, low-calorie	1 serving	25	0	2	670	0	1.5	0.0	0	63%
Thousand Island	1 serving	250	1	10	570	0	24.0	35.0	4	83%
SANDWICH										
chicken	1 sandwich	420	16	39	950	2	23.0	40.0	4	48%
chicken, 'Jack's Spicy'	1 sandwich	570	24	52	1020	2	29.0	50.0	3	46%
'Chicken Fajita Pita'	1 sandwich	280	24	25	840	3	9.0	75.0	4	29%

Food Name	Serv. Size	Total Cal.	Prot. gms	Carbs gms	Sod. mgs	Fiber gms	Fat gms	Chol. mgs	Sat.Fat gms	%Fat Cal.
chicken fillet, grilled	1 sandwich	480	27	39	1110	4	24.0	65.0	6	45%
'Chicken Supreme'	1 sandwich	830	33	67	2130	3	48.0	75.0	7	52%
'Philly Cheesesteak'	1 sandwich	580	33	56	1860	1	16.0	80.0	8	29%
'Sourdough Breakfast'	1 sandwich	450	21	36	1040	2	24.0	205.0	8	49%
SIDE DISH										
eggroll	3 egg rolls	440	15	40	1020	4	24.0	35.0	6	50%
french fries, curly, chili cheese	1 serving	650	14	60	1760	4	41.0	25.0	12	55%
french fries, curly, seasoned	1 serving	410	6	45	1010	4	23.0	0.0	5	50%
french fries, jumbo	1 serving	430	4	58	890	4	20.0	0.0	5	42%
french fries, regular	1 serving	350	4	46	710	3	16.0	0.0	4	42%
french fries, super scoop	1 serving	610	6	82	1250	5	28.0	0.0	6	42%
hash browns	1 serving	170	1	14	250	1	12.0	0.0	2	64%
jalapeños, stuffed	7 jalapeños	530	14	46	1730	3	31.0	60.0	12	54%
onion rings	1 serving	410	6	45	1010	4	23.0	0.0	5	50%
potato, bacon cheddar wedges	1 serving	800	20	49	1470	4	58.0	55.0	16	65%
TACO										
monster	1 serving	270	12	19	670	4	17.0	30.0	6	55%
regular	1 serving	170	7	12	460	2	10.0	20.0	4	54%
KENTUCKY FRIED CHICKEN										
BISCUIT	1 biscuit	180	4	20	560	0	10.0	0.0	3	48%
CHICKEN										
breast, extra crispy, w/o bone, 5.9 oz	1 breast	470	39	17	874	1	28.0	160.0	8	53%
breast, hot and spicy, w/o bone, 6.5 oz	1 breast	505	38	23	1170	1	29.0	162.0	8	52%
breast, original recipe, w/o bone, 5.4 oz	1 breast	400	29	16	1116	1	24.0	135.0	6	55%
drumstick, extra crispy, w/o bone, 2.4 oz	1 drumstick	195	15	7	375	1	12.0	77.0	3	55%
drumstick, hot and spicy, w/o bone, 2.3 oz	1 drumstick	175	13	9	360	1	10.0	77.0	3	51%
drumstick, original recipe, w/o bone, 2.2 oz	1 drumstick	140	13	4	422	0	9.0	75.0	2	54%
popcorn, large	6.0 oz	620	30	36	1046	0	40.0	73.0	10	58%
popcorn, small	3.5 oz	362	17	21	610	0	23.0	43.0	6	58%
thigh, extra crispy, w/o bone, 4.2 oz	1 thigh	380	21	14	625	1	27.0	118.0	7	63%
thigh, hot and spicy, w/o bone, 3.8 oz	1 thigh	355	19	13	630	1	26.0	126.0	7	65%
thigh, original recipe, w/o bone, 3.2 oz	1 thigh	250	16	6	747	1	18.0	95.0	5	65%
wing, honey barbecue	6 pieces	607	33	33	1145	1	38.0	193.0	10	56%
wing, hot	6 pieces	471	27	18	1230	2	33.0	150.0	8	62%
wing, whole, extra crispy, w/o bone, 1.9 oz	1 wing	220	10	10	415	1	15.0	55.0	4	63%
wing, whole, hot and spicy, w/o bone, 1.9 oz	1 wing	210	10	9	360	1	15.0	55.0	4	64%
wing, whole, original recipe, w/o bone, 1.6 oz	1 wing	140	9	5	414	0	10.0	55.0	3	62%
CHICKEN POT PIE, chunky	13 oz	770	29	69	2160	5	42.0	70.0	13	49%
CHICKEN SANDWICH										
honey barbecue, w/sauce, 5.3 oz	1 sandwich	310	28	37	560	2	6.0	125.0	2	17%
original recipe, w/o sauce, 6.6 oz	1 sandwich	360	28	3	890	1	13.0	60.0	4	49%

Food Name	Serv. Size	Total Cal.	Prot. gms	Carbs gms	Sod. mgs	Fiber gms	Fat gms	Chol. mgs	Sat.Fat gms	%Fat Cal.
original recipe, w/sauce, 7.3 oz ..... 1 sandwich		450	29	33	940	2	22.0	70.0	5	44%
'Tender Roast' w/o sauce, 6.2 oz .... 1 sandwich		270	31	26	690	1	5.0	65.0	2	16%
'Tender Roast' w/sauce, 7.4 oz ..... 1 sandwich		350	32	23	880	1	15.0	75.0	3	38%
'Triple Crunch Zinger' w/o sauce, 6.2 oz .... 1 sandwich		390	25	39	650	2	15.0	50.0	5	35%
'Triple Crunch Zinger' w/sauce, 7.4 oz .... 1 sandwich		550	28	36	830	2	32.0	85.0	7	53%
'Triple Crunch' w/o sauce, 6.2 oz .... 1 sandwich		390	25	39	650	2	15.0	50.0	5	35%
'Triple Crunch' w/o sauce, 6.6 oz .... 1 sandwich		490	28	29	710	2	29.0	70.0	6	53%
CHICKEN STRIPS										
crispy .... 3 strips		300	26	18	1165	1	16.0	56.0	4	45%
crispy, spicy .... 3 strips		335	25	23	1140	1	15.0	70.0	4	41%
DESSERT										
apple pie, 4.0 oz .... 1 slice		310	2	44	280	0	14.0	0.0	3	41%
double chocolate chip, 2.7 oz .... 1 serving		320	4	41	230	1	16.0	55.0	4	44%
'Little Bucket Parfait' chocolate creme, 4.0 oz .... 1 serving		290	3	37	330	2	15.0	15.0	11	46%
'Little Bucket Parfait' fudge brownie, 3.5 oz .... 1 serving		280	3	44	190	1	10.0	145.0	4	32%
'Little Bucket Parfait' lemon creme, 4.5 oz .... 1 serving		410	7	62	290	4	14.0	20.0	8	31%
'Little Bucket Parfait' strawberry shortcake, 3.5 oz .... 1 serving		200	1	33	220	1	7.0	10.0	6	32%
pecan pie, 4.0 oz .... 1 slice		490	5	66	510	2	23.0	65.0	5	42%
strawberry creme pie, 2.7 oz .... 1 slice		280	4	32	130	2	15.0	15.0	8	48%
SIDE DISH										
barbecue baked beans .... 5.5 oz		190	6	33	760	6	3.0	5.0	1	15%
coleslaw .... 5 oz		232	2	26	284	3	13.5	8.0	2	52%
corn on the cob .... 5.7 oz		150	5	35	20	2	1.5	0.0	0	8%
macaroni and cheese .... 5.4 oz		180	7	21	860	2	8.0	10.0	3	39%
mashed potato, w/gravy .... 4.8 oz		120	1	17	440	2	6.0	1.0	1	43%
potato salad .... 5.6 oz		230	4	23	540	3	14.0	15.0	2	54%
potato wedges .... 4.8 oz		280	5	28	750	5	13.0	5.0	4	47%
KRYSTAL										
BREAKFAST										
bacon biscuit .... 3.6 oz		355	9	36	1055	0	20.0	14.0	5	50%
egg biscuit .... 4.8 oz		372	10	36	813	0	21.0	133.0	5	51%
gravy biscuit .... 8.2 oz		445	9	43	1306	0	26.0	13.0	5	53%
plain biscuit .... 3.2 oz		289	5	35	777	0	14.0	1.0	3	44%
sausage biscuit .... 4.3 oz		429	10	37	987	0	27.0	29.0	7	56%
'Sunriser' .... 3.6 oz		264	13	17	551	0	17.0	157.0	6	56%
CHEESEBURGER										
'Burger Plus' .... 7 oz		545	33	37	962	0	31.0	105.0	12	50%
double patty .... 1 serving		214	11	22	674	0	8.0	16.0	2	35%
regular .... 1 serving		189	11	16	456	0	10.0	30.0	4	45%
w/bacon .... 6.4 oz		583	36	34	935	0	35.0	114.0	14	53%
CHILI										
large .... 12-oz serving		322	17	33	1012	0	11.0	25.0	0	33%
regular .... 8-oz serving		214	11	22	674	0	8.0	16.0	0	35%

Food Name	Serv. Size	Total Cal.	Prot. gms	Carbs gms	Sod. mgs	Fiber gms	Fat gms	Chol. mgs	Sat.Fat gms	%Fat Cal.
CORN DOG, 'Corn Pup'	2.3 oz	214	6	17	566	0	14.0	24.0	6	58%
DESSERT										
apple pie	4.5 oz	320	3	45	420	0	14.0	0.0	4	40%
lemon meringue pie	4 oz	340	7	60	130	0	9.0	45.0	3	23%
pecan pie	4 oz	450	5	61	290	0	24.0	55.0	6	45%
DOUGHNUT										
plain	1.3 oz	100	1	17	130	0	9.0	6.0	2	53%
w/chocolate icing	1.8 oz	162	1	27	149	0	11.0	6.0	3	47%
w/vanilla icing	1.8 oz	148	1	29	130	0	9.0	6.0	2	40%
HAMBURGER										
'Big K'	7.3 oz	608	40	35	1281	0	36.0	125.0	14	52%
'Burger Plus'	6.4 oz	488	30	36	709	0	27.0	90.0	9	48%
double patty	4 oz serving	276	18	24	532	0	14.0	43.0	5	43%
small	2.2 oz serving	158	9	15	339	0	7.0	21.0	0	40%
HOT DOG										
'Chili Cheese Pup'	2.6 oz	203	8	15	623	0	13.0	24.0	5	56%
'Chili Pup'	2.5 oz	184	7	14	593	0	12.0	19.0	4	56%
plain	1.9 oz	164	6	14	469	0	10.0	15.0	4	53%
MILKSHAKE, chocolate	12.8 fl oz	271	8	41	175	0	10.0	32.0	5	31%
SANDWICH										
chicken, 6.4 oz	1 sandwich	392	21	44	707	0	16.0	33.0	0	36%
country ham, 4.5 oz	1 sandwich	379	15	36	1488	0	19.0	23.0	5	46%
SIDE DISH										
french fries, crisscut, 'Krys Kross'	2.6 oz	242	3	33	589	0	11.0	10.0	5	41%
french fries, crisscut, 'Krys Kross' w/cheese	3.6 oz	292	4	35	789	0	15.0	11.0	6	46%
french fries, regular, large	5 oz serving	615	5	111	191	0	17.0	15.0	8	25%
french fries, regular, medium	3.9 oz serving	474	4	86	147	0	13.0	12.0	6	25%
french fries, regular, small	2.8 oz serving	338	3	61	105	0	9.0	8.0	0	24%
LITTLE CAESARS										
BREAD, 'Crazy Bread'	1 serving	98	4	18	119	0	1.0	2.0	0	9%
CONDIMENTS, 'Crazy Sauce'	1 serving	63	3	11	360	0	1.0	0.0	0	14%
PIZZA										
'Baby Pan! Pan!'	1 serving	525	28	53	1180	0	22.0	60.0	0	38%
cheese, single slice, 2.2 oz	1 slice	170	9	20	285	0	6.0	10.0	0	32%
pepperoni combination, single slice	1 serving	190	10	20	340	1	7.0	15.0	0	34%
'Pizza! Pizza!!' large	1 serving	169	11	18	240	0	6.0	15.0	0	32%
'Pizza! Pizza!!' medium	1 serving	154	10	16	220	0	5.0	15.0	0	30%
'Pizza! Pizza!!' small	1 serving	138	9	14	200	0	5.0	15.0	0	33%
'Pizza! Pizza!!' square, large	1 serving	188	10	22	380	0	6.0	20.0	0	30%
'Pizza! Pizza!!' square, medium	1 serving	185	10	22	370	0	6.0	20.0	0	30%
PIZZA MEAL										
cheese pizza, hand-tossed, w/individual tossed salad	1 serving	600	30	73	1605	3	21.0	35.0	0	31%
vegetable pizza, w/individual tossed salad	1 serving	640	34	76	1715	4	22.0	40.0	0	31%
SALAD										
antipasto, w/low-calorie dressing	12-oz serving	170	10	12	1145	0	9.0	40.0	0	48%
Greek, w/low-calorie dressing	11-oz serving	140	8	8	1075	0	8.0	25.0	0	53%

Food Name	Serv. Size	Total Cal.	Prot. gms	Carbs gms	Sod. mgs	Fiber gms	Fat gms	Chol. mgs	Sat.Fat gms	%Fat Cal.
tossed, small	1 serving	37	2	7	85	0	1.0	0.0	0	20%
tossed, w/low-calorie dressing	11-oz serving	80	4	11	745	0	2.0	0.0	0	23%
SANDWICH										
ham and cheese	1 sandwich	520	28	55	1045	1	21.0	45.0	0	36%
submarine, Italian	1 sandwich	590	29	55	1230	2	28.0	60.0	0	43%
tuna melt	1 sandwich	700	34	58	825	1	37.0	65.0	0	48%
turkey	1 sandwich	450	24	49	1590	0	17.0	45.0	0	34%
vegetarian	1 sandwich	620	30	58	1000	1	30.0	55.0	0	43%

LONG JOHN SILVER'S

Food Name	Serv. Size	Total Cal.	Prot. gms	Carbs gms	Sod. mgs	Fiber gms	Fat gms	Chol. mgs	Sat.Fat gms	%Fat Cal.
CHICKEN										
batter-dipped, 2 oz	1 piece	120	8	11	400	3	6.0	15.0	2	42%
'FlavorBaked'	2.6 oz	110	19	1	600	1	3.0	55.0	1	25%
CLAMS, batter-dipped	3 oz	300	11	31	670	5	17.0	40.0	4	48%
CONDIMENTS. See also Salad Dressing.										
catsup	0.32 oz	10	0	2	110	0	0.0	0.0	0	0%
honey mustard sauce	0.42 oz	20	0	5	60	na	0.0	0.0	0	0%
malt vinegar	0.28 oz	0	0	0	15	na	0.0	0.0	0	0%
margarine	0.18 oz	35	0	0	35	na	4.0	0.0	1	100%
shrimp sauce	0.42 oz	15	0	3	180	na	0.0	0.0	0	0%
sour cream	1 oz	60	1	1	15	na	6.0	15.0	4	87%
sweet and sour sauce	0.42 oz	20	0	5	45	na	0.0	0.0	0	0%
tartar sauce	0.42 oz	35	0	5	35	na	1.5	0.0	na	40%
FISH										
batter-dipped, 2.98 oz	1 piece	170	11	12	470	5	11.0	30.0	3	52%
'Flavorbaked' 2.3 oz	1 piece	90	14	1	320	0	2.5	35.0	1	27%
SALAD										
garden	1 salad	45	3	9	25	4	0.0	0.0	0	0%
grilled chicken	1 salad	140	20	10	260	4	2.5	45.0	1	16%
ocean chef	1 salad	130	14	15	540	4	2.0	60.0	0	13%
side	4.3 oz	25	1	4	15	1	0.0	0.0	0	0%
SALAD DRESSING										
French, fat-free	1.5 oz	50	0	14	360	na	0.0	0.0	0	0%
Italian	1 oz	130	0	2	280	na	14.0	0.0	2	94%
ranch	1 oz	170	0	1	260	na	18.0	5.0	3	98%
ranch, nonfat	1.5 oz	50	2	13	380	na	0.0	0.0	0	0%
Thousand Island	1 oz	110	0	5	280	na	10.0	15.0	2	82%
SANDWICH										
chicken, 'Flavorbaked'	5.8 oz	290	24	27	970	2	10.0	60.0	2	31%
fish, 'Flavorbaked'	6 oz	320	23	28	930	2	14.0	55.0	7	38%
fish, batter-dipped, no sauce	5.4 oz	320	17	40	800	6	13.0	20.0	4	34%
fish, 'Ultimate'	6.4 oz	430	18	44	1340	3	21.0	35.0	7	43%
SHRIMP, batter-dipped, 0.4 oz	1 piece	35	1	2	95	0	2.5	10.0	1	65%
SIDE DISH										
baked potato	8 oz	210	4	49	10	3	0.0	0.0	0	0%
cheese sticks	1.6 oz	160	6	12	360	1	9.0	10.0	4	53%
coleslaw	3.4 oz	140	1	20	260	3	6.0	0.0	na	39%
corn cobbette, w/butter	3.3 oz	140	3	19	0	0	8.0	0.0	2	45%
corn cobbette w/o butter	3.05 oz	80	3	19	0	0	0.5	0.0	0	5%
french fries	3 oz	250	3	28	500	3	15.0	0.0	3	52%
green beans	3.5 oz	30	2	5	310	2	0.5	5.0	0	14%

Food Name	Serv. Size	Total Cal.	Prot. gms	Carbs gms	Sod. mgs	Fiber gms	Fat gms	Chol. mgs	Sat.Fat gms	%Fat Cal.
hushpuppy, 0.8 oz	1 piece	60	1	9	25	0	2.5	0.0	0	36%
rice pilaf	3 oz	140	3	26	210	1	3.0	0.0	1	19%

MAZZIO'S
CHICKEN PARMESAN, noodles chicken

Food Name	Serv. Size	Total Cal.	Prot. gms	Carbs gms	Sod. mgs	Fiber gms	Fat gms	Chol. mgs	Sat.Fat gms	%Fat Cal.
Parmesan	17.5 oz	590	39	68	1600	0	19.0	50.0	3	29%
FETTUCCINE ALFREDO, small	1 serving	440	14	34	680	0	28.0	55.0	16	57%
GARLIC BREAD, w/cheese	2 slices	700	21	74	1280	0	35.0	15.0	7	45%
LASAGNA, meat, small	1 serving	460	24	26	1370	0	25.0	95.0	10	53%
NACHOS, meat	4.5 oz	500	21	21	1200	0	37.0	75.0	17	66%
PIZZA										
cheese, deep pan	1 serving	350	17	42	620	0	8.0	15.0	0	23%
cheese, original, medium	2 slices	260	14	33	450	0	8.0	10.0	0	28%
cheese, thick crust	1 serving	220	13	22	440	0	9.0	15.0	0	37%
combination, deep pan, medium	1 slice	410	19	42	930	0	18.0	20.0	6	40%
combination, original, medium	1 slice	320	17	34	780	0	13.0	25.0	6	36%
'Light' medium	1 slice	240	10	30	460	0	8.0	20.0	4	31%
pepperoni, deep pan, medium	1 slice	380	18	38	740	0	17.0	25.0	6	41%
pepperoni, original, medium	1 slice	280	16	30	600	0	11.0	30.0	5	35%
sausage, deep pan, medium	1 slice	430	21	41	1040	0	21.0	25.0	8	43%
sausage, original, medium	1 slice	350	18	34	890	0	16.0	20.0	7	41%
SANDWICH										
barbecue beef and cheddar	1 sandwich	580	39	53	1260	0	24.0	95.0	11	37%
chicken and cheddar	1 sandwich	570	33	56	1350	0	24.0	70.0	8	38%
ham and cheese sandwich	1 sandwich	790	40	71	1900	0	39.0	85.0	13	44%
SPAGHETTI ENTRÉE, small	1 serving	290	11	39	800	0	10.0	5.0	0	31%

MCDONALD'S
BEVERAGE

Food Name	Serv. Size	Total Cal.	Prot. gms	Carbs gms	Sod. mgs	Fiber gms	Fat gms	Chol. mgs	Sat.Fat gms	%Fat Cal.
apple bran muffin, low-fat	1 serving	300	6	61	380	3	3.0	0.0	1	9%
chocolate shake, small	1 small	360	11	60	250	1	9.0	40.0	6	22%
'Coca-Cola Classic' medium	21 fl oz	310	0	58	20	0	0.0	0.0	0	0%
'Diet Coke' medium	21 fl oz	0	0	0	40	0	0.0	0.0	0	0%
English muffin	1 serving	140	4	25	210	1	2.0	0.0	0	13%
orange drink, 'Hi-C' medium	21 fl oz	240	0	64	40	0	0.0	0.0	0	0%
milk, 1%	8 fl oz	100	8	13	115	0	2.5	10.0	2	21%
orange juice	6 fl oz	80	0	20	20	0	0.0	0.0	0	0%
'Sprite' medium	21 fl oz	210	0	56	80	0	0.0	0.0	0	0%
strawberry shake, small	1 serving	360	11	60	180	0	9.0	40.0	6	22%
vanilla shake, small	1 serving	360	11	59	250	0	9.0	40.0	6	22%
BREAKFAST										
apple Danish	1 serving	340	5	47	340	2	15.0	20.0	3	39%
bacon, egg, and cheese biscuit	1 sandwich	540	21	36	1550	1	34.0	250.0	10	57%
biscuit, plain or buttermilk	1 serving	262	4	35	757	1	11.9	1.8	1	40%
breakfast burrito	1 serving	320	13	21	660	1	20.0	195.0	7	57%
cheese Danish	1 serving	400	7	45	400	2	21.0	40.0	5	48%
cinnamon roll	1 serving	390	6	50	310	2	18.0	65.0	5	42%
'Egg McMuffin'	1 sandwich	290	17	27	790	1	12.0	235.0	5	38%
ham, egg, and cheese bagel	1 sandwich	550	26	58	1490	9	23.0	255.0	8	38%
hash browns	1 serving	130	1	14	330	1	8.0	0.0	2	55%
hotcakes, plain	1 serving	340	9	58	630	3	8.0	20.0	2	21%

Food Name	Serv. Size	Total Cal.	Prot. gms	Carbs gms	Sod. mgs	Fiber gms	Fat gms	Chol. mgs	Sat.Fat gms	%Fat Cal.
hotcakes, w/margarine and syrup	1 serving	600	9	104	770	3	17.0	20.0	3	25%
sausage and egg biscuit	1 sandwich	550	18	35	1160	1	37.0	245.0	10	61%
sausage	1 serving	170	6	0	290	0	16.0	35.0	5	86%
sausage biscuit	1 sandwich	470	11	35	1080	1	31.0	35.0	9	60%
'Sausage McMuffin'	1 sandwich	360	13	26	740	1	23.0	45.0	8	57%
'Sausage w/Egg McMuffin'	1 sandwich	440	19	27	890	1	28.0	255.0	10	58%
scrambled eggs	2 eggs	160	13	1	170	0	11.0	425.0	4	64%
Spanish omelette bagel	1 sandwich	690	27	59	1560	10	38.0	275.0	14	50%
steak egg and cheese bagel	1 sandwich	660	36	57	1300	9	31.0	285.0	11	43%
CHEESEBURGER										
'Big Xtra!'	1 burger	810	29	52	1870	4	55.0	120.0	19	60%
'Quarter Pounder with Cheese'	1 burger	530	28	38	1310	2	30.0	95.0	13	51%
regular	1 burger	320	16	35	830	2	13.0	40.0	6	36%
CHICKEN NUGGETS										
'Chicken McNuggets'	4 pieces	190	10	13	360	1	11.0	35.0	3	52%
'Chicken McNuggets'	6 piece	290	15	20	540	2	17.0	55.0	4	52%
'Chicken McNuggets'	9 piece	430	23	29	810	2	25.0	80.0	5	52%
CONDIMENTS. See also Salad Dressing.										
barbecue sauce	1 pkg	45	0	10	250	0	0.0	0.0	0	0%
croutons, salad bar item	1 pkg	50	1	9	105	1	1.0	0.0	0	18%
honey	1 pkg	45	0	12	0	0	0.0	0.0	0	0%
honey mustard sauce	1 pkg	50	0	3	85	0	4.5	10.0	1	77%
hot mustard sauce	1 pkg	60	1	7	240	0	3.5	5.0	1	50%
mayonnaise, light	1 pkg	40	0	0	80	0	4.0	5.0	1	100%
sweet and sour sauce	1 pkg	50	0	11	140	0	0.0	0.0	0	0%
DESSERT										
apple pie, baked	1 serving	260	3	34	200	0	13.0	0.0	4	44%
chocolate chip cookie	1 serving	170	2	22	120	1	10.0	20.0	6	48%
ice cream cone, vanilla, reduced fat	1 serving	150	4	23	75	0	4.5	20.0	3	27%
'McDonaldland'	1 pkg	180	3	32	190	1	5.0	0.0	1	24%
'McFlurry' Butterfinger	1 serving	620	16	90	260	0	22.0	70.0	14	32%
'McFlurry' M&M's	1 serving	630	16	90	210	1	23.0	75.0	15	33%
'McFlurry' Nestlé Crunch	1 serving	630	16	89	230	0	24.0	75.0	16	34%
'McFlurry' Oreo	1 serving	570	15	82	280	0	20.0	70.0	12	32%
nut topping, for sundae	1 serving	40	2	2	55	0	3.5	0.0	0	66%
sundae, hot caramel	1 serving	360	7	61	180	0	10.0	35.0	6	25%
sundae, hot fudge	1 serving	340	8	52	170	1	12.0	30.0	9	31%
sundae, strawberry	1 serving	290	7	50	95	0	7.0	30.0	5	22%
HAMBURGER										
'Big Mac'	1 burger	570	26	45	1100	3	32.0	85.0	10	50%
'Big Xtra!'	1 burger	710	24	51	1400	4	46.0	95.0	15	58%
'Quarter Pounder'	1 burger	430	23	37	840	2	21.0	70.0	8	44%
regular	1 burger	270	13	35	600	2	8.0	30.0	4	27%
SALAD										
shaker, chef	1 salad	150	17	5	740	2	8.0	95.0	4	45%
shaker, garden	1 salad	100	7	4	120	2	6.0	75.0	3	55%
shaker, grilled chicken Caesar	1 salad	100	17	3	240	2	2.5	40.0	2	22%
SALAD DRESSING										
Caesar	1 pkg	150	2	5	390	0	13.0	15.0	3	81%
herb vinaigrette, nonfat	1 pkg	30	0	7	220	0	0.0	0.0	0	0%
honey mustard	1 pkg	150	1	13	290	0	11.0	15.0	2	64%

Food Name	Serv. Size	Total Cal.	Prot. gms	Carbs gms	Sod. mgs	Fiber gms	Fat gms	Chol. mgs	Sat.Fat gms	%Fat Cal.
ranch	1 pkg	170	0	2	480	0	18.0	10.0	3	95%
red ranch, reduced calorie	1 pkg	130	0	18	370	0	6.0	0.0	1	43%
Thousand Island	1 pkg	130	0	11	360	0	9.0	15.0	2	65%
SANDWICH										
chicken, crispy	1 sandwich	550	23	54	1180	2	27.0	50.0	5	44%
'Chicken McGrill'	1 sandwich	450	26	46	970	2	18.0	60.0	3	36%
'Chicken McGrill' w/o mayo	1 sandwich	340	26	45	890	2	7.0	50.0	2	18%
'Fillet-O-Fish'	1 sandwich	470	15	45	890	1	26.0	50.0	5	49%
SIDE DISH										
french fries, large	1 serving	540	8	68	350	6	26.0	0.0	5	43%
french fries, medium	1 serving	450	6	57	290	5	22.0	0.0	4	44%
french fries, small	1 serving	210	3	26	135	2	10.0	0.0	2	44%
french fries, super size	1 serving	610	9	77	390	7	29.0	0.0	5	43%

MRS. WINNER
BISCUIT

Food Name	Serv. Size	Total Cal.	Prot. gms	Carbs gms	Sod. mgs	Fiber gms	Fat gms	Chol. mgs	Sat.Fat gms	%Fat Cal.
	1 serving	245	4	45	503	0	5.0	0.0	0	19%
CHICKEN										
breast, fried, no skin	4 oz	280	23	14	480	0	15.0	115.0	0	48%
fillet, baked	1 serving	120	10	0	360	0	2.0	33.0	0	31%
leg, fried, no skin	1.7 oz	110	10	5	115	0	6.0	50.0	0	47%
HAM, country	1 serving	60	4	0	565	0	1.0	14.0	0	36%
ROLL, honey yeast	1 roll	200	8	35	290	0	4.0	7.0	0	17%
SALAD										
chicken	1 salad	583	9	39	875	0	8.0	3.0	0	27%
seafood	1 salad	553	5	41	756	0	9.0	4.0	0	31%
tossed	1 salad	6	1	1	439	0	0.0	1.0	0	0%
SANDWICH										
chicken, breaded	1 sandwich	203	19	12	1000	0	10.0	37.0	0	42%
chicken fillet	1 sandwich	379	12	45	541	0	7.0	28.0	0	22%
chicken salad	1 sandwich	313	10	33	599	0	6.0	1.0	0	24%
steak	1 sandwich	429	11	43	644	0	11.0	21.0	0	31%
SAUSAGE, patty	1 serving	200	6	0	400	0	10.0	8.0	0	79%
SIDE DISH										
coleslaw	1 serving	188	1	9	549	0	16.0	1.0	0	78%
french fries	1 serving	225	6	27	214	0	9.0	1.0	0	38%
mashed potato, w/gravy	1 serving	148	3	22	823	0	3.0	2.0	0	21%
potato wedges, oven roasted	1 serving	139	4	31	132	0	1.0	1.0	0	6%
STEAK ENTRÉE, country fried	1 serving	220	12	0	205	0	14.0	7.0	0	72%

PERKINS

Food Name	Serv. Size	Total Cal.	Prot. gms	Carbs gms	Sod. mgs	Fiber gms	Fat gms	Chol. mgs	Sat.Fat gms	%Fat Cal.
BROCCOLI, raw	4 oz	31	3	6	31	0	0.4	0.0	0	9%
CHICKEN ENTRÉE										
lemon pepper, w/rice pilaf, broccoli, salad	1 serving	620	59	60	1364	0	12.5	136.0	0	19%
FRUIT CUP, w/cantaloupe, honeydew, blueberries	4.5 oz serving	48	1	12	12	0	0.3	0.0	0	5%
HASH BROWNS	3 oz	101	2	17	28	0	2.6	0.0	0	24%
MUFFIN										
apple	1 muffin	543	9	76	728	0	24.0	95.0	0	39%

Food Name	Serv. Size	Total Cal.	Prot. gms	Carbs gms	Sod. mgs	Fiber gms	Fat gms	Chol. mgs	Sat.Fat gms	%Fat Cal.
banana nut	1 muffin	586	9	75	702	0	29.0	92.0	0	44%
blueberry	1 muffin	506	7	71	671	0	23.0	88.0	0	40%
bran	1 muffin	478	9	83	572	0	17.0	0.0	0	29%
carrot	1 muffin	560	7	88	780	0	23.0	81.0	0	35%
chocolate chocolate chip	1 muffin	546	10	73	629	0	26.0	83.0	0	41%
corn	1 muffin	683	12	121	1550	0	17.0	33.0	0	22%
cranberry nut	1 muffin	558	9	71	671	0	28.0	88.0	0	44%
oat bran	1 muffin	513	10	87	588	0	16.0	0.0	0	27%
plain	1 muffin	586	9	81	797	0	26.0	104.0	0	39%
plain, low-fat	1 muffin	495	12	111	802	0	1.2	5.0	0	2%
OMELET										
'Country Club'	1 serving	932	47	6	1134	1	79.1	1154.0	0	77%
'Country Club' w/3 oz hash browns	1 serving	1033	49	23	1162	1	81.7	1154.0	0	72%
'Deli Ham and Lotsa Cheese'	1 serving	962	53	8	1832	1	79.1	864.0	0	74%
'Deli Ham and Lotsa Cheese' w/3 oz hash browns	1 serving	1063	55	25	1860	1	81.7	864.0	0	70%
'Denver' w/fruit cup	1 serving	235	23	22	795	0	6.5	154.0	0	24%
'Everything'	1 serving	697	45	9	870	0	53.4	814.0	0	69%
'Everything' w/3 oz hash browns	1 serving	798	46	25	898	2	56.0	814.0	0	64%
'Granny's Country'	1 serving	941	43	7	786	1	81.5	810.0	0	79%
'Granny's Country' w/9 oz hash browns	1 serving	1245	48	57	869	1	89.2	810.0	0	66%
ham and cheese	1 serving	644	41	3	832	0	51.3	743.0	0	73%
ham and cheese, w/3 oz hash browns	1 serving	745	42	19	860	0	53.9	743.0	0	66%
mushroom and cheese	1 serving	687	32	5	925	1	59.9	744.0	0	79%
mushroom and cheese, w/3 oz hash browns	1 serving	788	34	22	953	1	62.5	744.0	0	72%
seafood, w/fruit cup	1 serving	271	29	28	595	0	5.7	197.0	0	19%
ORANGE ROUGHY ENTRÉE,										
w/rice pilaf, broccoli, salad	1 serving	467	33	60	1387	0	7.0	133.0	0	14%
PANCAKE										
buttermilk	3 pancakes	442	13	70	988	0	12.0	24.0	0	25%
'Harvest Grain' w/1.5 oz low-cal syrup	5 pancakes	473	11	93	1640	0	3.4	0.0	0	7%
'Short Stack Harvest Grain'	3 pancakes	268	7	56	1020	0	2.0	0.0	0	7%
PIE										
apple	1 slice	521	3	72	457	0	26.0	0.0	0	44%
apple, w/Equal sugar substitute	1 slice	420	3	55	371	0	24.0	0.0	0	48%
cherry	1 slice	571	4	84	702	0	26.0	0.0	0	40%
cherry, w/Equal sugar substitute	1 slice	425	4	55	513	0	24.0	0.0	0	48%
coconut cream	1 slice	437	6	56	488	0	33.0	5.0	0	55%
French silk	1 slice	551	4	59	478	0	37.0	53.0	0	57%
lemon meringue	1 slice	395	2	63	528	0	16.0	0.0	0	36%
peanut butter brownie	1 slice	455	9	44	436	0	35.0	29.0	0	60%
pecan	1 slice	669	7	106	670	0	26.0	17.0	0	34%
SALAD										
chef, mini	1 salad	214	23	7	643	0	11.0	55.0	0	45%
dinner, 'Lite and Healthy'	1 salad	103	3	15	496	0	2.1	0.0	0	21%

Food Name	Serv. Size	Total Cal.	Prot. gms	Carbs gms	Sod. mgs	Fiber gms	Fat gms	Chol. mgs	Sat.Fat gms	%Fat Cal.
SYRUP, low-calorie	1.5 oz	26	0	7	0	0	0.0	0.0	0	0%
TOAST, w/.5 oz margarine,										
grape jelly	0.75-oz slice	219	2	28	224	1	12.2	8.0	0	48%
VEGETABLE STIR-FRY, w/mixed										
vegetables	6 oz	49	3	10	23	0	0.4	0.0	0	6%
VEGETABLE SANDWICH										
stir-fry, on pita	1 sandwich	308	44	41	752	0	9.2	26.0	0	20%
stir-fry, on pita, w/coleslaw	1 sandwich	441	45	54	877	0	17.8	36.0	0	29%
stir-fry, on pita, w/coleslaw and										
pasta salad	1 sandwich	626	49	63	1395	0	32.5	37.0	0	40%
stir-fry, on pita, w/pasta salad	1 sandwich	493	48	50	1270	0	23.9	27.0	0	35%

PETER PIPER PIZZA
PIZZA
Beef

Food Name	Serv. Size	Total Cal.	Prot. gms	Carbs gms	Sod. mgs	Fiber gms	Fat gms	Chol. mgs	Sat.Fat gms	%Fat Cal.
express lunch	1 slice	165	9	21	257	0	5.0	13.0	0	27%
extra large	1 slice	280	15	36	446	0	8.0	20.0	0	26%
large	1 slice	296	15	39	482	0	8.0	20.0	0	25%
medium	1 slice	222	12	29	359	0	6.0	15.0	0	25%
small	1 slice	194	10	25	319	0	5.0	14.0	0	24%
Cheese										
express lunch pizza	1 pizza	608	32	83	609	0	16.0	47.0	0	24%
express lunch pizza	1 slice	152	8	21	152	0	4.0	12.0	0	24%
extra large	1 pizza	3078	160	437	3113	0	73.0	211.0	0	22%
extra large	1 slice	257	13	36	260	0	6.1	18.0	0	22%
large	1 pizza	2159	112	311	2176	0	49.4	140.0	0	21%
large	1 slice	270	14	39	271	0	6.2	18.0	0	21%
medium	1 pizza	1622	84	235	1614	0	37.0	105.0	0	21%
medium	1 slice	203	11	29	201	0	5.0	13.0	0	22%
small	1 pizza	1059	60	152	1073	0	25.0	70.0	0	21%
small	1 slice	177	9	25	179	0	4.0	12.0	0	21%
w/black olive, large	1 slice	259	24	22	407	0	8.0	12.0	0	28%
w/black olive, medium	1 slice	193	18	17	303	0	6.0	9.0	0	28%
w/black olive, small	1 slice	171	16	15	276	0	6.0	8.0	0	30%
w/green pepper, large	1 slice	245	24	22	339	0	7.0	12.0	0	26%
w/green pepper, medium	1 slice	183	18	17	256	0	5.0	9.0	0	24%
w/green pepper, small	1 slice	163	16	15	283	0	4.0	8.0	0	23%
w/ham, large	1 slice	258	26	22	473	0	7.0	17.0	0	25%
w/ham, medium	1 slice	194	19	16	356	0	6.0	13.0	0	28%
w/ham, small	1 slice	172	17	15	317	0	5.0	11.0	0	26%
w/jalapeño, large	1 slice	244	24	22	424	0	7.0	12.0	0	26%
w/jalapeño, medium	1 slice	183	18	17	319	0	5.0	9.0	0	24%
w/jalapeño, small	1 slice	163	16	15	283	0	4.0	8.0	0	23%
w/mushroom, large	1 slice	245	24	22	379	0	7.0	12.0	0	26%
w/mushroom, medium	1 slice	183	18	17	283	0	5.0	9.0	0	24%
w/mushroom, small	1 slice	162	16	15	245	0	4.0	8.0	0	23%
w/onion, large	1 slice	243	24	22	341	0	7.0	12.0	0	26%
w/onion, medium	1 slice	183	18	17	257	0	5.0	9.0	0	24%
w/onion, small	1 slice	162	16	15	228	0	4.0	8.0	0	23%
w/pineapple, large	1 slice	246	23	23	341	0	7.0	12.0	0	26%

Food Name	Serv. Size	Total Cal.	Prot. gms	Carbs gms	Sod. mgs	Fiber gms	Fat gms	Chol. mgs	Sat.Fat gms	%Fat Cal.
w/pineapple, medium	1 slice	185	18	17	256	0	5.0	8.0	0	24%
w/pineapple, small	1 slice	164	16	15	228	0	4.0	8.0	0	23%
Salami										
express lunch	1 slice	164	9	21	199	0	5.0	15.0	0	27%
extra large	1 slice	273	14	37	322	0	7.5	22.0	0	25%
large	1 slice	288	15	39	342	0	8.0	23.0	0	25%
medium	1 slice	216	11	29	254	0	6.0	17.0	0	25%
small	1 slice	189	8	25	223	0	5.0	15.0	0	25%

PIZZA HUT

Food Name	Serv. Size	Total Cal.	Prot. gms	Carbs gms	Sod. mgs	Fiber gms	Fat gms	Chol. mgs	Sat.Fat gms	%Fat Cal.
BREADSTICK	1 serving	130	3	20	170	1	4.0	0.0	1	28%
BREADSTICK DIPPING SAUCE	1 serving	30	1	5	170	1	0.5	0.0	0	16%
CHICKEN										
Buffalo wings, hot	4 pieces	210	22	4	900	0	12.0	130.0	3	51%
Buffalo wings, mild	5 pieces	200	23	1	510	0	12.0	150.0	4	53%
GARLIC BREAD	1 slice	150	3	16	240	1	8.0	0.0	2	49%
PASTA										
cavatini	1 serving	480	21	66	1170	9	14.0	8.0	6	27%
'Cavatini Supreme'	1 serving	560	24	73	1400	10	19.0	10.0	8	31%
spaghetti, w/marinara sauce	1 serving	490	18	91	730	8	6.0	0.0	1	11%
spaghetti, w/meat sauce	1 serving	600	23	98	910	9	13.0	8.0	5	19%
spaghetti, w/meatballs	1 serving	850	37	120	1120	10	24.0	17.0	10	26%
PIZZA										
Apple, dessert	1 slice	250	3	48	230	2	4.5	0.0	1	17%
Beef										
hand-tossed, medium	1 slice	347	16	44	943	4	12.0	21.0	6	31%
pan, medium	1 slice	399	15	45	773	4	18.0	20.0	7	40%
Sicilian, medium	1 slice	282	13	31	824	3	12.0	19.0	7	38%
stuffed crust, medium	1 slice	466	23	46	1137	3	22.0	30.0	10	42%
thin and crispy, medium	1 slice	305	14	28	814	3	15.0	24.0	7	45%
Cheese										
'Big New Yorker'	1 slice	393	20	42	1099	3	16.6	18.5	8	38%
hand-tossed, medium	1 slice	309	14	43	848	3	9.0	11.0	5	26%
pan, medium	1 slice	361	13	44	678	3	15.0	11.0	6	37%
pan, personal	1 pizza	813	31	110	1581	8	27.0	24.0	12	30%
Sicilian, medium	1 slice	295	12	32	815	3	13.0	11.0	7	40%
stuffed crust, medium	1 slice	445	22	46	1090	3	19.0	24.0	10	39%
thin and crispy, medium	1 slice	243	11	27	653	2	10.0	11.0	5	37%
Cherry, dessert	1 slice	250	3	47	220	3	4.5	0.0	1	17%
'Chicken Supreme'										
hand-tossed, medium	1 slice	291	15	44	841	4	6.0	17.0	3	19%
pan, medium	1 slice	343	15	45	671	3	12.0	16.0	4	31%
Sicilian, medium	1 slice	269	13	32	732	3	10.0	15.0	5	33%
stuffed crust, medium	1 slice	432	24	47	1111	3	17.0	32.0	8	35%
'The New Edge' medium	1 slice	90	7	9	290	1	3.5	15.0	2	33%
thin and crispy, medium	1 slice	232	13	29	681	3	7.0	19.0	3	27%
Ham										
hand-tossed, medium	1 slice	279	13	43	857	3	6.0	15.0	3	19%
pan, medium	1 slice	331	12	44	687	3	12.0	15.0	4	33%
Sicilian, medium	1 slice	257	11	30	745	3	10.0	14.0	5	35%

Food Name	Serv. Size	Total Cal.	Prot. gms	Carbs gms	Sod. mgs	Fiber gms	Fat gms	Chol. mgs	Sat.Fat gms	%Fat Cal.
stuffed crust, medium	1 slice	404	24	45	1190	2	22.0	39.0	12	42%
thin and crispy, medium	1 slice	212	10	27	662	2	7.0	15.0	3	30%
Italian sausage
hand-tossed, medium	1 slice	363	16	44	975	4	14.0	26.0	6	34%
pan, medium	1 slice	415	15	45	805	3	20.0	26.0	7	43%
Sicilian, medium	1 slice	333	13	31	855	3	18.0	24.0	7	48%
stuffed crust, medium	1 slice	478	22	46	1164	3	23.0	35.0	10	43%
thin and crispy, medium	1 slice	325	14	28	865	3	18.0	32.0	7	49%
'Meat Lover's'
hand-tossed, medium	1 slice	376	17	44	1077	4	15.0	30.0	6	36%
pan, medium	1 slice	428	16	45	607	3	21.0	29.0	7	44%
Sicilian, medium	1 slice	344	14	31	948	3	18.0	27.0	8	47%
stuffed crust, medium	1 slice	543	26	46	1427	3	29.0	48.0	13	48%
'The New Edge' medium	1 slice	160	7	8	440	1	11.0	20.0	5	62%
thin and crispy, medium	1 slice	339	15	28	970	3	19.0	35.0	8	50%
Pepperoni
'Big New Yorker'	1 slice	380	18	42	1116	3	16.0	22.4	7	38%
hand-tossed, medium	1 slice	301	13	43	867	3	8.0	15.0	4	24%
pan, medium	1 slice	353	12	44	697	3	14.0	14.0	5	36%
pan, personal	1 pizza	810	30	111	1661	8	28.0	32.0	11	31%
Sicilian, medium	1 slice	227	11	31	754	3	113.0	13.0	5	86%
stuffed crust, medium	1 slice	438	21	45	1116	2	19.0	27.0	9	39%
thin and crispy, medium	1 slice	235	10	27	672	2	10.0	14.0	4	38%
'Pepperoni Lover's'
hand-tossed, medium	1 slice	372	17	43	1123	3	14.0	26.0	7	34%
pan, medium	1 slice	370	13	44	767	3	16.0	18.0	5	39%
Sicilian, medium	1 slice	321	13	31	899	3	16.0	19.0	8	45%
stuffed crust, medium	1 slice	525	26	46	1413	3	26.0	40.0	13	45%
thin and crispy, medium	1 slice	289	13	28	859	2	14.0	22.0	6	43%
Pork
hand-tossed, medium	1 slice	342	16	44	990	4	12.0	20.0	5	31%
pan, medium	1 slice	394	15	45	820	4	18.0	20.0	6	40%
Sicilian, medium	1 slice	314	13	31	868	3	16.0	18.0	7	45%
stuffed crust, medium	1 slice	461	22	46	1176	3	21.0	29.0	10	41%
thin and crispy, medium	1 slice	298	14	28	875	3	15.0	23.0	6	45%
'Super Supreme'
hand-tossed, medium	1 slice	359	16	45	1024	4	12.0	23.0	5	31%
pan, medium	1 slice	401	15	46	854	4	18.0	22.0	6	40%
Sicilian, medium	1 slice	323	13	32	911	3	16.0	21.0	7	44%
stuffed crust, medium	1 slice	505	25	46	1371	3	25.0	44.0	11	44%
thin and crispy, medium	1 slice	304	14	29	902	3	15.0	26.0	6	44%
'Supreme'
'Big New Yorker'	1 slice	459	10	44	1310	4	22.3	33.2	9	48%
hand-tossed, medium	1 slice	333	15	44	927	4	11.0	18.0	5	30%
pan, medium	1 slice	385	14	45	757	4	17.0	18.0	6	39%
pan, personal	1 pizza	808	30	111	1579	8	27.0	28.0	10	30%
Sicilian, medium	1 slice	307	13	32	815	3	15.0	17.0	7	43%
stuffed crust, medium	1 slice	487	24	47	1227	3	23.0	33.0	11	42%
thin and crispy, medium	1 slice	284	13	29	784	3	13.0	20.0	6	41%

Food Name	Serv. Size	Total Cal.	Prot. gms	Carbs gms	Sod. mgs	Fiber gms	Fat gms	Chol. mgs	Sat.Fat gms	%Fat Cal.
Taco										
beef, hand-tossed, medium	1 slice	270	13	35	870	3	8.0	15.0	4	27%
beef, pan, medium	1 slice	300	12	36	770	3	12.0	15.0	5	36%
beef, thin and crispy, medium	1 slice	260	13	29	850	2	10.0	20.0	5	35%
chicken, hand-tossed, medium	1 slice	290	12	35	940	3	11.0	15.0	5	34%
chicken, pan, medium	1 slice	320	12	36	830	3	15.0	15.0	5	41%
chicken, thin and crispy, medium	1 slice	260	11	26	850	2	12.0	20.0	5	42%
hand-tossed, medium	1 slice	280	12	34	870	3	11.0	15.0	5	35%
meatless, hand-tossed, medium	1 slice	250	11	35	790	3	8.0	10.0	4	28%
meatless, pan, medium	1 slice	290	10	36	680	3	12.0	10.0	4	37%
meatless, thin and crispy, medium	1 slice	230	9	27	700	2	8.0	10.0	4	33%
pan, medium	1 slice	310	12	36	800	3	13.0	15.0	5	38%
pan, personal	1 pizza	780	27	90	1900	7	35.0	30.0	10	40%
thin and crispy, medium	1 slice	260	12	27	860	2	11.0	20.0	5	39%
'The Works' 'The New Edge' medium	1 slice	110	5	9	270	1	6.0	10.0	3	49%
'Veggie Lover's'										
hand-tossed, medium	1 slice	281	12	45	771	4	6.0	7.0	3	19%
pan, medium	1 slice	333	11	46	601	4	12.0	7.0	4	32%
Sicilian, medium	1 slice	252	10	32	627	3	10.0	7.0	5	35%
stuffed crust, medium	1 slice	421	20	48	1039	3	17.0	19.0	8	36%
'The New Edge' medium	1 slice	70	4	9	180	1	3.0	5.0	2	34%
thin and crispy, medium	1 slice	222	9	30	621	3	8.0	7.0	3	32%
SANDWICH										
ham and cheese	1 sandwich	550	33	57	2150	4	21.0	22.0	7	34%
'Supreme'	1 sandwich	640	34	62	2150	4	28.0	28.0	10	40%
PONDEROSA										
CHICKEN ENTRÉE										
breast	5.5 oz	98	20	1	400	0	2.1	54.0	0	19%
wing	2 pieces	213	11	11	610	0	9.0	75.0	0	49%
CONDIMENTS. See also Salad Bar Items; Salad Dressing.										
cheese sauce	2 oz	52	1	6	355	0	2.0	4.0	0	37%
cheese topping, herb and garlic	1 tbsp	100	0	0	120	0	10.0	0.0	0	100%
gravy, brown	2 oz	25	1	4	167	0	1.0	0.0	0	33%
gravy, turkey	2 oz	25	1	5	228	0	0.2	0.0	0	7%
margarine, liquid	1 tbsp	100	0	0	110	0	11.0	0.0	0	100%
margarine, whipped	1 tbsp	34	0	0	65	0	1.2	0.0	0	100%
tartar sauce	1 oz	85	0	11	477	0	10.9	9.0	0	69%
DESSERT										
dougnut, winter mix	3.5 oz	25	2	4	371	0	0.0	0.0	0	0%
gelatin dessert, plain, nonfat	4 oz	71	1	17	73	0	0.0	0.0	0	0%
ice milk, chocolate	3.5 oz	152	4	30	70	0	3.0	22.0	0	17%
ice milk, vanilla	3.5 oz	150	4	30	58	0	3.0	20.0	0	17%
mousse, chocolate	4 oz	312	0	28	72	0	18.0	0.0	0	59%
mousse, chocolate	1 oz	78	0	7	18	0	4.4	0.0	0	59%
mousse, strawberry	4 oz	297	0	25	68	0	18.0	0.0	0	62%
mousse, strawberry	1 oz	74	0	6	17	0	4.6	0.0	0	62%
pudding, banana	4 oz	207	1	27	114	0	10.0	0.0	0	45%
vanilla wafer cookie, peanut butter	2 wafers	35	0	6	25	0	1.0	5.0	0	27%

Food Name	Serv. Size	Total Cal.	Prot. gms	Carbs gms	Sod. mgs	Fiber gms	Fat gms	Chol. mgs	Sat.Fat gms	%Fat Cal.
DESSERT TOPPING										
caramel	1 oz	100	0	26	72	0	0.7	2.0	0	6%
chocolate	1 oz	89	1	24	37	0	0.3	0.0	0	3%
peanut, granulated	.2 oz	30	1	1	0	0	2.3	0.0	0	69%
strawberry	1 oz	71	0	24	29	0	0.2	0.0	0	2%
strawberry glaze	1 oz	37	0	10	4	0	0.0	0.0	0	0%
whipped	1 oz	80	0	5	16	0	7.0	0.0	0	76%
FISH. See also individual listings.										
nuggets	1 piece	31	2	2	52	0	1.7	8.0	0	52%
baked, 'Bake 'R Broil' baked	5.2 oz	230	19	10	330	0	13.0	50.0	0	50%
fried	3.2 oz	190	9	17	170	0	9.0	15.0	0	44%
HALIBUT, broiled	6 oz	170	35	0	68	0	2.4	0.0	0	13%
HOT DOG	1.6 oz	144	5	1	460	0	13.0	27.0	0	83%
MEATBALLS	2 pieces	115	5	2	16	0	4.0	21.0	0	56%
ORANGE ROUGHY, broiled	5 oz	139	0	21	88	0	5.0	28.0	0	35%
ROLL										
dinner	1 piece	184	5	33	311	0	3.0	0.0	0	15%
sourdough	1 piece	110	4	22	230	0	1.0	0.0	0	8%
SALAD BAR ITEMS										
banana chips	.2 oz	25	0	3	0	0	1.3	0.0	0	46%
banana	1 medium	87	1	23	1	0	0.2	0.0	0	2%
breadstick, Italian	1 stick	100	4	19	200	0	1.0	0.0	0	9%
breadstick, sesame	2 sticks	35	1	6	60	0	0.0	0.0	0	0%
broccoli, raw	1 oz	9	1	2	4	0	0.0	0.0	0	43%
cabbage, green	1 oz	9	1	2	7	0	0.0	0.0	0	0%
cheese, imitation, shredded	1 oz	90	6	1	420	0	7.0	5.0	0	69%
chicken macaroni salad	3.5 oz	335	8	49	431	0	12.0	9.0	0	32%
chicken salad	3.5 oz	212	11	8	334	0	15.0	42.0	0	64%
chow mein noodles	.2 oz	25	1	3	42	0	1.2	0.0	0	43%
coconut, shredded	.2 oz	25	0	2	14	0	1.9	0.0	0	66%
croutons	1 oz	115	4	18	351	0	4.0	0.0	0	29%
fruit cocktail	4 oz	97	1	25	7	0	0.2	0.0	0	2%
granola	.2 oz	24	1	3	0	0	1.0	0.0	0	38%
grapes	10 grapes	34	0	9	2	0	0.2	0.0	0	5%
ham, diced	2 oz	120	9	1	780	0	10.0	76.0	0	69%
lemon	1 wedge	3	0	1	0	0	0.1	0.0	0	20%
macaroni salad	3.5 oz	335	8	49	431	0	11.7	9.0	0	32%
onion, green	1 piece	7	0	2	1	0	0.1	0.0	0	11%
onion, yellow	1 oz	11	0	3	3	0	0.0	0.0	0	0%
orange	1 piece	45	1	11	1	0	0.1	0.0	0	2%
pasta salad	3.5 oz	268	6	34	441	0	12.0	0.0	0	40%
pickle chips, sweet	.14 oz	4	0	1	1	0	0.0	0.0	0	0%
pickle spear, dill	.14 oz	1	0	0	54	0	0.0	0.0	0	0%
potato salad	3.5 oz	126	2	16	300	0	6.0	7.0	0	43%
turkey ham salad	3.5 oz	186	8	10	654	0	13.0	12.0	0	62%
turkey, julienne	1 oz	29	5	1	192	0	1.0	15.0	0	27%
yogurt, frozen, fruit flavor	4 oz	115	5	23	70	0	1.0	5.0	0	7%
yogurt, frozen, vanilla	4 oz	110	5	18	75	0	2.0	6.0	0	16%
SALAD DRESSING										
blue cheese	1 oz	130	1	1	266	0	14.0	27.0	0	94%

Food Name	Serv. Size	Total Cal.	Prot. gms	Carbs gms	Sod. mgs	Fiber gms	Fat gms	Chol. mgs	Sat.Fat gms	%Fat Cal.
coleslaw	1 oz	150	0	6	284	0	14.0	31.0	0	84%
creamy Italian	1 oz	103	0	3	373	0	10.0	0.0	0	88%
cucumber, lower calorie	1 oz	69	0	3	315	0	6.0	0.0	0	82%
Italian, lower calorie	1 oz	31	0	1	371	0	3.0	0.0	0	87%
oil	1 tbsp	120	0	0	0	0	14.0	0.0	0	100%
Parmesan pepper	1 oz	150	1	2	281	0	15.0	9.0	0	92%
ranch	1 oz	147	0	1	297	0	15.0	3.0	0	97%
sweet-n-tangy	1 oz	122	0	8	347	0	10.0	1.0	0	74%
Thousand Island	1 oz	113	0	8	405	0	10.0	9.0	0	74%
SALMON, broiled	6 oz	192	37	3	72	0	3.0	60.0	0	14%
SCROD, baked	7 oz	120	27	0	80	0	1.0	65.0	0	8%
SHRIMP										
fried	7 pieces	230	22	31	612	0	1.0	105.0	0	4%
mini	6 pieces	47	5	6	125	0	1.0	22.0	0	17%
SIDE DISH										
baked beans	4 oz	170	6	21	330	0	6.0	0.0	0	33%
baked potato	7.2 oz	145	4	33	6	0	0.0	0.0	0	0%
corn	3.5 oz	90	3	21	5	0	0.4	0.0	0	4%
french fries	3 oz	120	2	17	39	0	4.0	3.0	0	32%
green beans	3.5 oz	20	1	3	391	0	0.0	0.0	0	0%
macaroni and cheese	1 oz	17	1	4	80	0	0.5	1.0	0	18%
macaroni salad	3.5 oz	335	8	49	431	0	11.7	9.0	0	32%
mashed potato	4 oz	62	2	13	191	0	0.0	20.0	0	0%
okra, breaded	4 oz	124	3	23	483	0	1.0	1.0	0	8%
onion rings, breaded	4 oz	213	3	30	620	0	9.0	2.0	0	38%
pasta/noodles	2 oz	78	2	16	1	0	0.3	0.0	0	4%
potato wedges	3.5 oz	130	3	16	170	0	6.0	0.0	0	42%
rice pilaf	4 oz	160	4	26	450	0	4.0	22.0	0	23%
spinach	1 oz	7	1	1	20	0	0.1	0.0	0	10%
stuffing	4 oz	230	6	27	800	0	11.0	22.0	0	43%
SPAGHETTI, w/sauce	6 oz	188	5	33	520	0	5.0	0.0	0	23%
STEAK										
chopped	4 oz	225	19	1	150	0	16.0	80.0	0	64%
kabobs, meat only	3 oz	153	26	2	280	0	5.0	67.0	0	29%
Kansas City strip	5 oz	138	21	1	850	0	5.7	76.0	0	37%
New York strip, choice	8 oz	314	45	1	570	0	10.5	50.0	0	34%
Porterhouse, choice	16 oz	640	57	3	1130	0	30.9	82.0	0	54%
Porterhouse, non-graded	13 oz	440	43	1	1844	0	30.0	67.0	0	61%
ribeye, choice	6 oz	282	29	1	570	0	14.0	60.0	0	51%
ribeye, non-graded	5 oz	219	25	1	1130	0	13.0	75.0	0	53%
sirloin, choice	7 oz	241	35	1	570	0	11.0	63.0	0	41%
sirloin tips, choice	5 oz	197	29	1	280	0	8.0	71.0	0	38%
T-bone, choice	10 oz	444	44	2	850	0	18.0	80.0	0	47%
T-bone, non-graded	8 oz	178	25	2	850	0	8.5	71.0	0	42%
teriyaki	5 oz	174	32	5	1420	0	3.0	64.0	0	15%
STEAK SANDWICH	4 oz	208	20	2	850	0	11.0	62.0	0	53%
SWORDFISH, broiled	5.9 oz	271	44	0	0	0	10.0	84.0	0	34%
TROUT	5 oz	228	30	1	51	0	4.0	110.0	0	23%

POPEYES

Food Name	Serv. Size	Total Cal.	Prot. gms	Carbs gms	Sod. mgs	Fiber gms	Fat gms	Chol. mgs	Sat.Fat gms	%Fat Cal.
BISCUIT, plain or buttermilk	1 biscuit	233	4	31	673	1	10.6	1.6	1	40%

Food Name	Serv. Size	Total Cal.	Prot. gms	Carbs gms	Sod. mgs	Fiber gms	Fat gms	Chol. mgs	Sat.Fat gms	%Fat Cal.
CHICKEN										
breast, mild, w/o bone	3.7 oz	270	23	9	660	2	15.9	60.0	0	53%
breast, spicy, w/o bone	3.7 oz	270	23	9	590	2	15.9	60.0	0	53%
leg, mild, w/o bone	1.7 oz	120	10	4	240	0	7.3	40.0	0	53%
leg, spicy, w/o bone	1.7 oz	120	10	4	240	0	7.3	40.0	0	53%
nuggets, fried	4.2 oz	410	17	18	660	3	31.9	55.0	0	67%
thigh, mild, w/o bone	3.1 oz	300	15	9	620	1	22.7	70.0	0	68%
thigh, spicy, w/o bone	3.1 oz	300	15	9	450	1	22.7	70.0	0	68%
wing, mild, w/o bone	1.6 oz	160	9	7	290	0	10.7	40.0	0	60%
wing, spicy, w/o bone	1.6 oz	160	9	7	290	0	10.7	40.0	0	60%
DESSERT										
apple pie	3.1 oz	290	3	37	820	2	15.8	10.0	0	48%
SHRIMP	2.8 oz	250	16	13	650	3	16.4	110.0	0	56%
SIDE DISH										
Cajun rice	3.9 oz	150	10	17	1260	3	5.4	25.0	0	31%
coleslaw	4 oz	149	1	14	271	3	11.2	3.0	0	63%
corn on the cob	5.2 oz	90	4	21	20	9	2.9	0.0	0	20%
french fries	3 oz	240	4	31	610	3	12.2	10.0	0	44%
mashed potato, w/gravy	3.8 oz	100	5	11	460	3	6.0	5.0	0	47%
onion rings	3.1 oz	310	5	31	210	2	19.3	25.0	0	55%
red beans and rice	5.9 oz	270	8	30	680	7	16.9	10.0	0	51%
QUINCY'S										
CATFISH, fillet, 2 pieces	6.9-oz serving	309	26	19	101	0	12.0	0.0	0	38%
CHEESEBURGER, 1/4 lb										
precooked	1 serving	451	28	32	432	0	23.0	0.0	0	46%
CHICKEN										
breast, grilled	5-oz serving	145	35	0	140	0	0.4	72.0	0	3%
strips, 4 pieces	4.5 oz	318	39	4	0	0	15.0	0.0	0	44%
CHILI, w/beans	9.2-oz serving	346	20	32	1380	0	16.0	0.0	0	41%
CORNBREAD	1.9-oz serving	178	4	28	263	0	6.0	0.0	0	30%
HAMBURGER, 1/4 lb precooked	1 serving	403	25	32	284	0	19.0	0.0	0	43%
MUSHROOM SAUCE	3-oz serving	27	1	5	366	0	1.0	0.0	0	27%
SHRIMP, 7 pieces	3.9-oz serving	248	22	11	205	0	12.0	0.0	0	45%
SIDE DISH										
baked potato, w/o butter	8.8-oz serving	181	5	41	8	0	1.0	0.0	0	5%
coleslaw	2.1-oz serving	60	1	4	75	0	5.0	0.0	0	69%
green beans	4.3-oz serving	40	2	7	500	0	1.0	0.0	0	20%
peppers and onions	4-oz serving	80	1	8	11	0	5.0	0.0	0	56%
steak fries	5.5-oz serving	426	7	56	90	0	21.0	0.0	0	43%
SOUP										
broccoli, cream of	9.2-oz serving	193	3	13	1045	0	14.0	0.0	0	66%
clam chowder	9.2-oz serving	198	6	15	1185	0	14.0	0.0	0	60%
vegetable beef soup	8.6-oz serving	78	5	10	1045	0	2.0	0.0	0	23%
STEAK										
chopped, luncheon	4-oz serving	350	30	0	72	0	25.0	0.0	0	65%
country style, w/mushroom										
sauce	6-oz serving	288	18	17	315	0	19.0	0.0	0	55%
fillet	5.6-oz serving	331	51	0	159	0	12.0	0.0	0	35%
ribeye	7.3-oz serving	665	31	0	205	0	60.0	0.0	0	81%

Food Name	Serv. Size	Total Cal.	Prot. gms	Carbs gms	Sod. mgs	Fiber gms	Fat gms	Chol. mgs	Sat.Fat gms	%Fat Cal.
sirloin	5.9-oz serving	649	38	0	206	0	54.0	0.0	0	76%
sirloin club	4.8-oz serving	283	44	0	160	0	10.0	0.0	0	34%
sirloin tips	4-oz serving	236	37	0	113	0	9.0	0.0	0	35%
sirloin, large	7.7-oz serving	852	50	0	241	0	70.0	0.0	0	76%
sirloin, petite	4-oz serving	446	26	0	118	0	37.0	0.0	0	76%
T-bone	7.8-oz serving	1045	43	0	222	0	95.0	0.0	0	83%

RALLY'S
CHEESEBURGER

Food Name	Serv. Size	Total Cal.	Prot. gms	Carbs gms	Sod. mgs	Fiber gms	Fat gms	Chol. mgs	Sat.Fat gms	%Fat Cal.
'Bacon Cheeseburger'	1 burger	622	33	35	1629	0	40.3	99.0	0	57%
'Double Cheeseburger'	1 burger	733	42	34	1473	0	49.1	92.0	0	59%
'Rallyburger w/Cheese'	1 burger	486	24	33	1185	0	29.4	79.0	0	53%
CHEESEBURGER MEAL										
'Large Combo' w/soft drink	1 meal	1018	29	129	1645	0	45.0	89.0	0	39%
'Small Combo' w/soft drink	1 meal	764	33	85	1416	0	37.2	84.0	0	42%
CHICKEN SANDWICH	1 sandwich	531	18	40	364	0	30.8	18.0	0	55%
CHILI	8 oz	340	22	21	1199	0	19.0	67.0	0	50%
FRENCH FRIES										
large	1 serving	317	5	39	439	0	15.6	10.0	0	44%
regular	1 serving	158	3	20	219	0	7.8	5.0	0	44%
HAMBURGER 'Rallyburger'	1 burger	436	21	33	955	0	24.9	67.0	0	51%
HAMBURGER MEAL										
'Large Combo' w/soft drink	1 meal	968	26	129	1415	0	40.5	76.0	0	37%
'Small Combo' w/soft drink	1 meal	714	24	84	1186	0	32.7	71.0	0	41%
SAUSAGE										
'Smokin' Sausage'	1 serving	724	28	31	1998	0	55.0	40.0	0	68%
'Smokin' Sausage' w/chili	1 serving	830	35	35	2163	0	62.0	67.0	0	67%
TACO, soft	1 taco	223	12	17	377	0	9.9	36.0	0	43%

RAX

Food Name	Serv. Size	Total Cal.	Prot. gms	Carbs gms	Sod. mgs	Fiber gms	Fat gms	Chol. mgs	Sat.Fat gms	%Fat Cal.
BEEF, roast beef	2.8 oz	140	14	1	524	0	9.0	36.0	0	57%
BREADSTICK, sesame, salad bar item	1 oz	150	3	13	405	0	10.0	0.0	0	58%
CHEESE, American, processed, slices	0.5 oz	60	3	1	180	0	5.0	15.0	0	74%
CONDIMENTS. See also SALAD DRESSING.										
Alfredo sauce, pasta bar item	3.5 oz	80	2	12	70	0	3.0	10.0	0	33%
banana pepper, Mexican bar item	1 tbsp	2	1	1	20	0	1.0	0.0	0	53%
barbecue meat topping	3.25 oz	140	13	13	898	0	4.0	24.0	0	26%
celery, salad bar item	1 tbsp	1	1	1	10	0	1.0	0.0	0	53%
cheese sauce, regular, Mexican bar item	3.5 oz	420	10	58	365	0	17.0	11.0	0	36%
chili topping	3 oz	80	8	8	221	0	2.0	18.0	0	22%
chow mein noodles, salad bar item	1 oz	140	4	17	242	0	6.0	1.0	0	39%
coconut, salad bar item	1 oz	160	1	15	1	0	11.0	0.0	0	61%
croutons, salad bar item	0.5 oz	40	2	8	155	0	1.0	1.0	0	18%
green onion, Mexican bar item	1/4 cup	10	1	2	1	0	1.0	0.0	0	43%
margarine, liquid	1 tbsp	100	1	1	100	0	11.0	0.0	0	93%
mushroom sauce	1 oz	16	1	1	113	0	1.0	0.0	0	53%
nacho cheese sauce, Mexican bar item	3.5 oz	470	10	57	190	0	22.0	11.0	0	42%
onion, diced	0.5 oz	10	1	1	1	0	1.0	0.0	0	53%

Food Name	Serv. Size	Total Cal.	Prot. gms	Carbs gms	Sod. mgs	Fiber gms	Fat gms	Chol. mgs	Sat.Fat gms	%Fat Cal.
pickle	1 spear	8	1	2	928	0	1.0	0.0	0	43%
sour topping	3.5 oz	130	3	5	79	0	11.0	1.0	0	76%
spaghetti sauce, pasta bar item	3.5 oz	80	1	19	635	0	1.0	1.0	0	10%
spaghetti sauce, w/meat, pasta bar item	3.5 oz	150	7	12	419	0	8.0	1.0	0	49%
spicy meat sauce, Mexican bar item	3.5 oz	80	5	6	751	0	4.0	12.0	0	45%
sunflower seeds and raisins, salad bar item	1 oz	130	5	6	5	0	10.0	0.0	0	67%
taco sauce, Mexican bar item	3.5 oz	30	1	6	806	0	1.0	0.0	0	24%
taco shell, Mexican bar item	1 shell	40	1	6	53	0	2.0	0.0	0	39%
turkey bits, salad bar item	2 oz	70	10	1	686	0	3.0	49.0	0	38%
DESSERT										
butterscotch pudding, salad bar item	3.5 oz	141	2	20	151	0	6.0	2.0	0	38%
chocolate chip cookie	1 cookie	130	1	17	65	0	6.0	1.0	0	43%
chocolate pudding, salad bar item	3.5 oz	141	2	20	121	0	6.0	2.0	0	38%
lime gelatin, salad bar item	1/2 cup	90	2	20	90	0	1.0	0.0	0	9%
strawberry gelatin, salad bar item	1/2 cup	90	2	20	90	0	1.0	0.0	0	9%
vanilla pudding, salad bar item	3.5 oz	141	2	20	121	0	6.0	2.0	0	38%
DESSERT TOPPING, whipped	1 dollop	50	1	4	6	0	4.0	2.0	0	64%
PASTA										
rainbow rotini, pasta bar item	3.5 oz	180	6	30	9	0	4.0	2.0	0	20%
shells, pasta bar item	3.5 oz	170	7	27	2	0	4.0	0.0	0	21%
spaghetti, pasta bar item	3.5 oz	140	3	23	1	0	4.0	0.0	0	26%
vegetable, pasta bar item	3.5 oz	100	4	12	11	0	4.0	0.0	0	36%
SALAD										
chef, w/o dressing	12.5-oz serving	230	22	4	1048	0	14.0	322.0	0	55%
garden, gourmet, 'Lighterside'	1 serving	134	7	13	350	0	6.0	2.0	0	40%
garden, w/o dressing	10.5-oz serving	160	12	4	362	0	11.0	273.0	0	61%
SALAD DRESSING										
blue cheese	1 tbsp	50	1	1	110	0	5.0	8.0	0	85%
blue cheese, 'Lite'	1 tbsp	35	1	2	240	0	3.0	3.0	0	69%
French	1 tbsp	60	1	6	140	0	4.0	0.0	0	56%
Italian	1 tbsp	50	1	3	159	0	4.0	0.0	0	69%
Italian, 'Lite'	1 tbsp	30	1	1	152	0	3.0	0.0	0	77%
oil	1 tbsp	130	1	1	1	0	14.0	0.0	0	94%
poppyseed	1 tbsp	60	1	5	107	0	4.0	6.0	0	60%
ranch	1 tbsp	45	1	1	103	0	5.0	5.0	0	85%
Thousand Island	1 tbsp	70	1	6	110	0	6.0	8.0	0	66%
Thousand Island, 'Lite'	1 tbsp	40	1	3	143	0	3.0	5.0	0	63%
vinegar	1 tbsp	2	1	1	5	0	1.0	0.0	0	53%
SANDWICH										
barbecue	5.7-oz serving	420	21	53	1343	0	14.0	24.0	0	30%
beef, bacon, and chicken, 'BBC'	8-oz serving	720	30	40	1873	0	49.0	137.0	0	61%
fish	7-oz serving	460	14	58	935	0	17.0	1.0	0	35%
ham and Swiss	7.9-oz serving	430	23	42	1737	0	23.0	37.0	0	44%
Philly beef and cheese	8.25-oz serving	480	25	44	1346	0	22.0	49.0	0	42%
roast beef, large	8-oz serving	570	22	41	1169	0	35.0	36.0	0	56%
roast beef, regular	5.25-oz serving	320	20	33	969	0	11.0	36.0	0	32%
roast beef, 'Uncle Al' small	3.1-oz serving	260	12	21	562	0	14.0	19.0	0	49%
turkey bacon club	9-oz serving	670	29	41	1878	0	43.0	87.0	0	58%

Food Name	Serv. Size	Total Cal.	Prot. gms	Carbs gms	Sod. mgs	Fiber gms	Fat gms	Chol. mgs	Sat.Fat gms	%Fat Cal.
SIDE DISH										
baked potato, barbecue, w/2 oz cheese	1 serving	730	24	104	1071	0	24.0	18.0	0	30%
baked potato, cheese and bacon	3-oz serving	780	22	110	910	0	28.0	23.0	0	32%
baked potato, cheese and broccoli	3-oz serving	760	19	112	489	0	26.0	11.0	0	31%
baked potato, chili, w/2 oz cheese	1 serving	700	22	101	599	0	23.0	25.0	0	30%
baked potato, plain	8.8-oz serving	270	8	60	70	0	1.0	0.0	0	3%
baked potato, w/margarine	9.3-oz serving	370	8	60	170	0	11.0	0.0	0	27%
baked potato, w/sour cream topping	1 serving	400	11	65	149	0	11.0	0.0	0	25%
broccoli, salad bar item	1/2 cup	16	2	2	7	0	1.0	0.0	0	36%
coleslaw, salad bar item	3.5 oz	70	1	8	187	0	4.0	1.0	0	50%
french fries, large, salted	4.5-oz serving	390	3	50	104	0	20.0	16.0	0	46%
french fries, large, unsalted	4.5-oz serving	390	3	50	66	0	20.0	16.0	0	46%
french fries, regular, salted	3-oz serving	260	2	33	69	0	13.0	10.0	0	46%
french fries, regular, unsalted	3-oz serving	260	2	33	44	0	13.0	10.0	0	46%
grapefruit sections, salad bar item	1 cup	80	2	18	10	0	1.0	0.0	0	10%
grapes, salad bar item	1 cup	100	1	25	5	0	1.0	0.0	0	8%
kale, salad bar item	1 oz	16	2	2	21	0	1.0	0.0	0	36%
kidney beans, salad bar item	1 cup	220	14	40	8	0	1.0	0.0	0	4%
macaroni salad, salad bar item	3.5 oz	160	2	21	216	0	7.0	1.0	0	41%
pasta salad, salad bar item	3.5 oz	80	2	16	322	0	1.0	1.0	0	11%
potato salad, salad bar item	1 cup	260	7	41	0	0	7.0	7.0	0	25%
refried beans, Mexican bar item	3 oz	120	6	16	375	0	4.0	2.0	0	29%
Spanish rice, Mexican bar item	3.5 oz	90	3	20	442	0	1.0	0.0	0	9%
three-bean salad	1/2 cup	100	3	23	450	0	1.0	0.0	0	8%
SOUP										
broccoli, cream of	3.5 oz	50	1	6	219	0	2.0	1.0	0	39%
chicken soup w/noodles, pasta bar item	3.5 oz	40	2	8	1040	0	1.0	10.0	0	18%
RED LOBSTER										
CALAMARI										
breaded, fried dinner portion	10 oz	720	26	60	2300	0	42.0	280.0	12	52%
breaded, fried, lunch portion	5 oz	360	13	30	1150	0	21.0	140.0	6	52%
CATFISH										
dinner portion	10 oz	340	40	0	100	0	20.0	170.0	6	53%
lunch portion	5 oz	170	20	0	50	0	10.0	85.0	3	53%
CHICKEN, breast	4-oz serving	120	24	0	60	0	3.0	65.0	1	22%
CLAMS										
cherrystone, dinner portion	10 oz	260	36	22	1080	0	4.0	160.0	0	13%
cherrystone, lunch portion	5 oz	130	18	11	540	0	2.0	80.0	0	13%
COD										
Atlantic, fillet, dinner portion	10 oz	200	46	0	400	0	2.0	140.0	0	9%
Atlantic, fillet, lunch portion	5 oz	100	23	0	200	0	1.0	70.0	0	9%
CRAB										
king, legs, 1 lb.	1 serving	170	32	6	900	0	2.0	100.0	0	11%
snow, legs, 1 lb.	1 serving	150	33	1	1630	0	2.0	130.0	1	12%
FLOUNDER										
dinner portion	10 oz	200	42	2	190	0	2.0	140.0	0	9%

Food Name	Serv. Size	Total Cal.	Prot. gms	Carbs gms	Sod. mgs	Fiber gms	Fat gms	Chol. mgs	Sat.Fat gms	%Fat Cal.
lunch portion	5 oz	100	21	1	95	0	1.0	70.0	0	9%
GROUPER										
dinner portion	10 oz	220	52	0	140	0	2.0	130.0	0	8%
lunch portion	5 oz	110	26	0	70	0	1.0	65.0	0	8%
HADDOCK										
dinner portion	10 oz	220	48	4	360	0	2.0	170.0	0	8%
lunch portion	5 oz	110	24	2	180	0	1.0	85.0	0	8%
HALIBUT										
dinner portion	10 oz	220	50	2	210	0	2.0	120.0	0	8%
lunch portion	5 oz	110	25	1	105	0	1.0	60.0	0	8%
HAMBURGER, 1/3 lb before cooked	1 serving	320	27	0	70	0	23.0	105.0	11	66%
LANGOSTINO										
dinner portion	10 oz	240	52	4	820	0	2.0	420.0	0	7%
lunch portion	5 oz	120	26	2	410	0	1.0	210.0	0	7%
LOBSTER										
Maine, cooked, 1-1/4 lb	1 serving	240	36	5	550	0	8.0	310.0	2	31%
rock, tail, cooked	1 serving	230	49	2	1090	0	3.0	200.0	1	12%
MACKEREL										
dinner portion	10 oz	380	2	40	500	0	24.0	200.0	8	56%
raw weight	5 oz	190	1	20	250	0	12.0	100.0	4	56%
MONKFISH										
dinner portion	10 oz	220	0	48	190	0	2.0	160.0	0	9%
lunch portion	5 oz	110	0	24	95	0	1.0	80.0	0	9%
MUSSELS	3-oz serving	70	9	3	150	0	2.0	50.0	0	27%
OCEAN PERCH										
Atlantic, dinner portion	10 oz	260	48	2	380	0	8.0	150.0	2	26%
Atlantic, lunch portion	5 oz	130	24	1	190	0	4.0	75.0	1	26%
OYSTERS, on half shell	6 oysters	110	8	11	90	0	4.0	60.0	2	32%
POLLACK										
dinner portion	10 oz	240	56	2	180	0	2.0	180.0	0	7%
lunch portion	5 oz	120	28	1	90	0	1.0	90.0	0	7%
RED ROCKFISH										
dinner portion	10 oz	180	42	0	190	0	2.0	170.0	0	10%
lunch portion	5 oz	90	21	0	95	0	1.0	85.0	0	10%
RED SNAPPER										
dinner portion	10 oz	220	50	0	280	0	2.0	140.0	0	8%
lunch portion	5 oz	110	25	0	140	0	1.0	70.0	0	8%
SALMON										
Norwegian, dinner portion	10 oz	460	54	6	120	0	24.0	160.0	6	47%
Norwegian, lunch portion	5 oz	230	27	3	60	0	12.0	80.0	3	47%
sockeye, dinner portion	10 oz	320	56	6	120	0	8.0	100.0	2	23%
sockeye, lunch portion	5 oz	160	28	3	60	0	4.0	50.0	1	23%
SCALLOPS										
calico, dinner portion	10 oz	360	64	16	320	0	4.0	230.0	0	10%
calico, lunch portion	5 oz	180	32	8	260	0	2.0	115.0	0	10%
deep sea, dinner portion	10 oz	260	52	4	520	0	4.0	100.0	0	14%
deep sea, lunch portion	5 oz	130	26	2	260	0	2.0	50.0	0	14%
SHARK										
blacktip, dinner portion	10 oz	300	70	0	180	0	2.0	120.0	0	6%

Food Name	Serv. Size	Total Cal.	Prot. gms	Carbs gms	Sod. mgs	Fiber gms	Fat gms	Chol. mgs	Sat.Fat gms	%Fat Cal.
blacktip, lunch portion	5 oz	150	35	0	90	0	1.0	60.0	0	6%
mako, dinner portion	10 oz	280	68	0	120	0	2.0	200.0	0	6%
mako, lunch portion	5 oz	140	34	0	60	0	1.0	100.0	0	6%
SHRIMP, 8–12 pieces	1 serving	120	25	0	110	0	2.0	230.0	0	15%
SOLE										
w/lemon, dinner portion	10 oz	240	54	2	180	0	2.0	130.0	0	7%
w/lemon, lunch portion	5 oz	120	27	1	90	0	1.0	65.0	0	7%
STEAK, strip	7 oz	690	29	0	70	0	64.0	140.0	27	83%
SWORDFISH										
dinner portion	10 oz	200	34	0	280	0	8.0	200.0	2	35%
lunch portion	5 oz	100	17	0	140	0	4.0	100.0	1	35%
TILEFISH										
dinner portion	10 oz	200	40	0	120	0	4.0	160.0	2	18%
lunch portion	5 oz	100	20	0	60	0	2.0	80.0	1	18%
TROUT										
rainbow, dinner portion	10 oz	340	46	0	180	0	18.0	180.0	6	47%
rainbow, lunch portion	5 oz	170	23	0	90	0	9.0	90.0	3	47%
TUNA										
yellowfin, dinner portion	10 oz	360	64	0	140	0	12.0	140.0	4	30%
yellowfin, lunch portion	5 oz	180	32	0	70	0	6.0	70.0	2	30%

ROUND TABLE
PIZZA

Food Name	Serv. Size	Total Cal.	Prot. gms	Carbs gms	Sod. mgs	Fiber gms	Fat gms	Chol. mgs	Sat.Fat gms	%Fat Cal.
'Alfredo Contempo'										
pan crust	1 slice	220	12	27	240	1	7.4	25.0	4	30%
thin crust	1 slice	170	9	17	210	1	6.5	25.0	4	36%
'Bacon Super Deli'										
pan crust	1 slice	260	12	26	380	0	13.5	25.0	5	44%
thin crust	1 slice	200	9	16	360	0	12.6	25.0	5	53%
Cheese										
pan	1 slice	210	10	26	250	1	7.2	20.0	5	31%
thin crust	1 slice	170	8	17	330	1	5.6	25.0	4	34%
Chicken and garlic										
pan, gourmet	1 slice	230	11	27	310	1	8.1	25.0	4	32%
thin crust, gourmet	1 slice	170	9	17	280	0	7.2	25.0	4	38%
'Classic Pesto'										
pan	1 slice	230	9	27	240	1	8.8	15.0	4	35%
thin crust	1 slice	170	7	18	210	1	7.9	15.0	4	42%
'Garden Delight'										
pan crust	1 slice	200	9	27	250	1	6.2	15.0	4	28%
thin crust	1 slice	150	7	18	250	1	5.6	15.0	3	34%
'Garden Pesto'										
pan crust	1 slice	230	9	28	230	1	8.6	15.0	4	34%
thin crust	1 slice	170	7	18	200	1	7.7	15.0	4	41%
'Gourmet Veggie'										
pan crust	1 slice	220	9	28	230	1	7.4	20.0	4	31%
thin crust	1 slice	160	7	18	200	1	6.5	15.0	3	37%
Italian Garlic Supreme'										
pan crust	1 slice	250	10	27	240	1	10.5	25.0	4	39%
thin crust	1 slice	200	8	17	220	0	10.4	25.0	4	48%

Food Name	Serv. Size	Total Cal.	Prot. gms	Carbs gms	Sod. mgs	Fiber gms	Fat gms	Chol. mgs	Sat.Fat gms	%Fat Cal.
'King Arthur's Supreme'										
pan crust	1 slice	240	10	27	320	1	9.8	25.0	4	37%
thin crust	1 slice	200	9	18	340	1	10.1	25.0	4	46%
Pepperoni										
pan crust	1 slice	220	9	26	240	1	8.1	20.0	4	34%
thin crust	1 slice	170	8	17	240	0	8.0	20.0	3	42%
'Salute Chicken Cashew'										
pan crust	1 slice	200	9	31	260	1	4.5	15.0	2	20%
thin crust	1 slice	150	7	21	240	1	4.1	15.0	2	25%
'Salute Chicken and Garlic'										
pan crust	1 slice	200	9	28	270	1	5.8	20.0	3	26%
thin crust	1 slice	150	8	18	250	1	5.4	20.0	3	32%
'Salute Veggie'										
pan crust	1 slice	190	8	28	190	1	5.1	10.0	3	24%
thin crust	1 slice	140	6	19	170	1	4.7	10.0	2	30%
'Santa Fe Chicken'										
pan crust	1 slice	240	11	27	360	1	9.2	30.0	5	35%
thin crust	1 slice	180	9	17	310	1	7.8	25.0	4	40%

ROY ROGERS

Food Name	Serv. Size	Total Cal.	Prot. gms	Carbs gms	Sod. mgs	Fiber gms	Fat gms	Chol. mgs	Sat.Fat gms	%Fat Cal.
BISCUIT	1 serving	231	4	26	575	0	12.0	5.0	0	47%
BREAKFAST										
apple swirl Danish	1 serving	328	5	62	279	0	7.0	0.0	0	19%
cheese swirl Danish	1 serving	383	8	54	369	0	15.0	0.0	0	35%
cinnamon rod pastry,	1 serving	376	5	55	339	0	15.0	0.0	0	36%
crescent, regular	1 serving	408	13	28	820	0	27.0	207.0	0	60%
crescent, w/bacon	1 serving	446	15	28	982	0	30.0	212.0	0	61%
crescent, w/ham	1 serving	456	20	29	1243	0	29.0	227.0	0	57%
crescent, w/sausage	1 serving	564	19	28	1145	0	42.0	248.0	0	67%
egg platter, w/bacon and biscuit	1 serving	607	21	44	1236	0	39.0	424.0	0	57%
egg platter, w/biscuit, regular	1 serving	557	18	44	1020	0	34.0	417.0	0	55%
egg platter, w/ham and biscuit,	1 serving	605	25	44	1442	0	36.0	437.0	0	54%
egg platter, w/sausage and biscuit	1 serving	713	25	44	1345	0	49.0	458.0	0	62%
pancake platter, regular, w/syrup and butter, regular	1 serving	386	5	63	547	0	13.0	51.0	0	30%
pancake platter, w/bacon, w/syrup and butter	1 serving	436	8	63	763	0	17.0	58.0	0	35%
pancake platter, w/ham, w/syrup and butter	1 serving	434	11	64	969	0	15.0	71.0	0	31%
pancake platter, w/sausage, w/syrup and butter	1 serving	542	11	63	872	0	28.0	92.0	0	46%
CHEESEBURGER										
'Express'	1 serving	613	30	42	1122	0	37.0	82.0	0	54%
'Express' w/bacon	1 serving	641	33	36	1317	0	41.0	89.0	0	57%
regular	1 serving	525	29	37	830	0	29.0	76.0	0	50%
regular, w/bacon	1 sandwich	520	24	32	1620	na	33.0	72.0	18	57%
small	1 serving	275	15	24	558	0	13.0	36.0	0	43%
CHICKEN										
breast, fried	1 serving	412	33	17	609	0	24.0	118.0	0	52%
breast and wing, fried	1 serving	604	44	25	894	0	37.0	165.0	0	55%

Food Name	Serv. Size	Total Cal.	Prot. gms	Carbs gms	Sod. mgs	Fiber gms	Fat gms	Chol. mgs	Sat.Fat gms	%Fat Cal.
breast and wing, w/o skin, 'Roy's Roaster'	1 serving	190	32	2	0	0	6.0	0.0	0	28%
dark meat, 1/4 'Roy's Roaster'	1 serving	490	43	2	1120	0	34.0	225.0	10	63%
dark meat, w/o skin, 1/4 'Roy's Roaster'	1 serving	190	24	1	400	0	10.0	110.0	3	47%
leg, fried	1 serving	140	12	6	190	0	8.0	40.0	0	50%
leg and thigh, fried	1 serving	436	30	17	596	0	28.0	125.0	0	57%
nuggets, fried, 9 pieces	9 pieces	435	18	30	915	na	27.0	22.5	6	56%
nuggets, fried, 6 pieces	6 pieces	290	12	20	610	na	18.0	15.0	4	56%
thigh, fried	1 serving	296	18	12	406	0	20.0	85.0	0	60%
white meat, 1/4 'Roy's Roaster'	1 serving	500	56	3	1450	0	29.0	240.0	9	53%
white meat, w/o skin, '1/4 Roy's Roaster'	1 serving	190	32	2	700	0	6.0	100.0	2	28%
wing, fried	1 serving	192	11	9	285	0	13.0	47.0	0	59%
CONDIMENTS. See also Salad Dressing.										
Chinese noodles, salad bar item	1/4 cup	55	2	7	113	0	3.0	1.0	0	43%
croutons, salad bar item	2 tbsp	14	1	3	50	0	0.0	0.0	0	0%
granola, salad bar item	1/4 cup	65	2	9	8	0	3.0	0.0	0	38%
grapes, salad bar item	5 grapes	20	0	5	1	0	0.0	0.0	0	0%
onion, chopped, salad bar item	2 tbsp	7	0	2	0	0	0.0	0.0	0	0%
DESSERT										
caramel sundae	1 serving	293	7	52	193	0	9.0	23.0	0	26%
chocolate sundae	1 serving	358	8	61	290	0	10.0	37.0	0	25%
gelatin parfait, salad bar item	1/4 cup	50	1	10	23	0	2.0	0.0	0	29%
hot fudge sundae	1 serving	337	7	53	186	0	13.0	23.0	0	33%
strawberry shortcake	1 serving	440	8	39	420	na	19.0	15.0	5	48%
strawberry sundae	1 serving	216	6	33	99	0	7.0	23.0	0	29%
vanilla sundae	1 serving	306	8	45	282	0	11.0	40.0	0	32%
HAMBURGER										
'Express'	1 serving	561	27	42	899	0	32.0	70.0	0	51%
regular	1 serving	472	26	37	607	0	25.0	64.0	0	47%
'Roy Rogers Bar'	1 serving	573	36	38	1252	0	31.0	96.0	0	49%
small	1 serving	222	12	23	336	0	9.0	26.0	0	37%
ROLL, crescent	1 serving	287	5	27	547	0	18.0	5.0	0	56%
SALAD, grilled chicken	1 salad	120	18	2	520	0	4.0	60.0	0	31%
SALAD DRESSING										
bacon and tomato	2 tbsp	136	0	6	150	0	12.0	0.0	0	82%
blue cheese	2 tbsp	150	2	2	153	0	16.0	0.0	0	90%
Italian, low-calorie	2 tbsp	70	0	2	100	0	6.0	0.0	0	87%
ranch	2 tbsp	155	0	4	100	0	14.0	0.0	0	89%
Thousand Island	2 tbsp	160	0	4	150	0	16.0	0.0	0	90%
SANDWICH										
chicken, 'Gold Rush'	1 sandwich	558	22	51	1326	na	30.0	35.0	9	48%
fish	1 sandwich	514	18	58	857	0	24.0	62.0	0	42%
roast beef	1 sandwich	329	31	29	875	na	10.0	62.0	3	27%
roast beef, large	1 sandwich	373	35	31	840	0	12.0	82.0	0	29%
roast beef, w/cheese	1 sandwich	403	29	37	954	0	15.0	70.0	0	34%
roast beef, w/cheese, large	1 sandwich	427	38	31	1062	0	17.0	94.0	0	36%
SIDE DISH										
baked potato, plain, 'Hot Topped'	1 serving	211	6	48	65	0	0.0	0.0	0	0%
broccoli, salad bar item	1/4 cup	6	1	1	6	0	0.0	0.0	0	0%

Food Name	Serv. Size	Total Cal.	Prot. gms	Carbs gms	Sod. mgs	Fiber gms	Fat gms	Chol. mgs	Sat.Fat gms	%Fat Cal.
coleslaw	1 serving	110	1	11	261	0	7.0	5.0	0	57%
french fries, large	5.5 oz serving	440	6	54	225	0	22.0	19.0	0	45%
french fries, regular	4 oz serving	320	4	39	164	0	16.0	13.0	0	46%
french fries, small	3 oz serving	238	3	29	122	0	12.0	10.0	0	46%
fruit cocktail, salad bar item	1/4 cup	46	0	12	1	0	0.0	0.0	0	0%
Greek noodles, salad bar item	1/4 cup	159	3	19	328	0	9.0	0.0	0	48%
lettuce, Romaine, salad bar item	1 cup	9	1	1	5	0	0.0	0.0	0	0%
macaroni salad, salad bar item	1/4 cup	93	2	10	301	0	5.0	0.0	0	48%
potato salad, salad bar item	1/4 cup	54	1	5	348	0	3.0	0.0	0	53%

SCHLOTZSKY'S DELI
BEVERAGE

Food Name	Serv. Size	Total Cal.	Prot. gms	Carbs gms	Sod. mgs	Fiber gms	Fat gms	Chol. mgs	Sat.Fat gms	%Fat Cal.
'Coca-Cola' regular	20 fl oz	248	na	68	15	na	0.0	na	na	0%
'Diet Coke' regular	20 fl oz	0	na	0	25	na	0.0	na	na	0%
iced tea, regular	20 fl oz	na	na	na	na	na	na	na	na	0%
lemonade, 'All Natural' regular	20 fl oz	183	na	43	14	0	0.0	0	0	0%
'Mr. Pibb' regular	20 fl oz	243	na	65	35	na	0.0	na	na	0%
orange, 'Minute Maid' regular	20 fl oz	265	na	73	0	na	0.0	na	na	0%
root beer, 'Barq's' regular	20 fl oz	278	na	75	60	na	0.0	na	na	0%
'Sprite' regular	20 fl oz	243	na	65	55	na	na	na	na	0%
CHILI, 'Timberline'	8 oz cup	210	14	24	814	7	7.0	32.0	3	29%

CONDIMENTS. See also Salad Dressing.

Food Name	Serv. Size	Total Cal.	Prot. gms	Carbs gms	Sod. mgs	Fiber gms	Fat gms	Chol. mgs	Sat.Fat gms	%Fat Cal.
croutons, garlic cheese, salad bar item	1 crouton	46	1	5	142	0	2.0	0.0	0	43%
chow mein noodles	1 serving	74	2	9	111	1	4.0	0.0	1	45%

DESSERT

Food Name	Serv. Size	Total Cal.	Prot. gms	Carbs gms	Sod. mgs	Fiber gms	Fat gms	Chol. mgs	Sat.Fat gms	%Fat Cal.
cookies and creme cheesecake	1 serving	330	6	36	320	1	18.0	35.0	9	49%
chocolate chip cookie	1 cookie	160	2	23	150	0	7.0	10.0	3	39%
chocolate chunk cookie	1 cookie	160	2	23	150	1	7.0	10.0	2	39%
chocolate pecan chunk cookie	1 cookie	170	2	23	140	1	8.0	10.0	2	42%
fudge brownie cake	1 serving	410	5	46	135	3	25.0	35.0	11	52%
fudge chocolate chunk cookie	1 cookie	170	2	22	170	1	8.0	10.0	3	43%
New York style cheesecake	1 serving	310	7	31	230	0	18.0	60.0	10	52%
oatmeal raisin cookie	1 cookie	150	2	1	na	na	1.0	200.0	10	43%
peanut butter cookie	1 cookie	170	2	21	190	1	8.0	10.0	2	44%
peanut butter chocolate cookie	1 cookie	170	2	21	160	1	8.0	10.0	3	44%
strawberry swirl cheesecake	1 serving	300	6	30	230	0	17.0	55.0	9	52%
sugar cookie	1 cookie	160	2	23	180	0	6.0	15.0	1	35%
white chocolate macadamia cookie	1 cookie	170	2	22	140	0	8.0	10.0	3	43%

PIZZA

Food Name	Serv. Size	Total Cal.	Prot. gms	Carbs gms	Sod. mgs	Fiber gms	Fat gms	Chol. mgs	Sat.Fat gms	%Fat Cal.
bacon, tomato, and mushroom, sourdough crust, 8-inch	1 pizza	635	27	78	1891	4	24.0	38.0	10	34%
barbecue chicken, sourdough crust, 8-inch	1 pizza	653	38	78	2103	3	20.0	74.0	9	28%
chicken and pesto, sourdough crust, 8-inch	1 pizza	649	40	78	2187	4	19.0	74.0	9	27%
double cheese and pepperoni, sourdough crust, 8-inch	1 pizza	744	32	77	2206	4	34.0	62.0	16	41%
double cheese, sourdough crust, 8-inch	1 pizza	603	26	77	1772	4	21.0	34.0	10	31%

Food Name	Serv. Size	Total Cal.	Prot. gms	Carbs gms	Sod. mgs	Fiber gms	Fat gms	Chol. mgs	Sat.Fat gms	%Fat Cal.
fresh tomato and pesto, sourdough										
crust, 8-inch	1 pizza	539	23	76	1670	4	16.0	27.0	8	27%
Mediterranean, sourdough crust,										
8-inch	1 pizza	564	24	84	1787	3	19.0	36.0	10	28%
New Orleans, sourdough crust, 8-inch	1 pizza	666	40	79	2493	4	20.0	74.0	9	27%
original combination, sourdough crust,										
8-inch	1 pizza	648	26	79	1994	5	25.0	41.0	10	35%
smoked turkey and jalapeño, sourdough										
crust, 8-inch	1 pizza	647	38	81	2591	4	19.0	62.0	8	26%
Southwestern, sourdough crust, 8-inch	1 pizza	635	38	76	2015	4	19.0	71.0	8	27%
Thai chicken, sourdough crust, 8-inch	1 pizza	681	40	88	2303	5	19.0	72.0	9	25%
vegetarian special, sourdough crust,										
8-inch	1 pizza	551	24	76	1757	4	17.0	27.0	8	28%
SALAD										
Caesar, w/o dressing, croutons, chow										
mein noodles	1 salad	152	11	11	505	4	8.0	15.0	4	45%
chef's, ham and turkey, dressing,										
croutons, chow mein noodles	1 salad	248	23	15	1442	3	11.0	51.0	5	39%
chef's, smoked turkey, w/o dressing,										
croutons, chow mein noodles	1 salad	243	24	15	1275	3	10.0	53.0	5	37%
chicken Caesar, w/o dressing,										
croutons, chow mein noodles	1 salad	254	28	13	935	4	10.0	63.0	5	35%
chicken, Chinese, w/o dressing,										
croutons, chow mein noodles	1 salad	150	20	11	448	3	3.0	47.0	1	18%
garden, small, w/o dressing, croutons,										
chow mein noodles	1 salad	25	1	3	55	1	1.0	0.0	0	36%
garden, w/o dressing, croutons, chow										
mein noodles	1 salad	61	3	8	119	3	1.0	0.0	0	17%
Greek, w/o dressing, croutons, chow										
mein noodles	1 salad	220	13	25	563	4	12.0	27.0	8	42%
SALAD DRESSING										
Caesar, 'Olde World'	1 pkt	260	2	1	250	0	27.0	25.0	5	95%
Greek balsamic vinaigrette	1 pkt	170	0	2	330	0	17.0	0.0	3	95%
Italian, light	1 pkt	90	0	3	690	0	8.0	0.0	2	86%
ranch, spicy	1 pkt	230	1	2	310	0	25.0	15.0	4	95%
ranch, spicy, light	1 pkt	140	1	9	350	0	11.0	15.0	3	71%
ranch, traditional	1 pkt	270	0	1	370	0	29.0	5.0	5	98%
sesame ginger vinaigrette	1 pkt	170	1	8	370	0	15.0	0.0	3	79%
Thousand Island	1 pkt	220	0	6	360	0	21.0	30.0	3	89%
SANDWICH										
Bacon, lettuce and tomato										
large, on sourdough bun	1 sandwich	1141	41	140	3066	6	46.0	80.0	14	36%
regular, on sourdough bun	1 sandwich	578	21	70	1548	3	24.0	41.0	7	37%
small, on sourdough bun	1 sandwich	379	13	47	1010	2	15.0	26.0	5	36%
Cheese										
large, on sourdough bun	1 sandwich	1857	87	159	4365	8	98.0	180.0	56	47%
regular, on sourdough bun	1 sandwich	854	38	79	2107	4	44.0	72.0	23	46%
small, on sourdough bun	1 sandwich	596	27	53	1432	3	31.0	54.0	17	47%
Chicken										
breast, large, on sourdough bun	1 sandwich	1008	72	158	4522	6	15.0	155.0	4	13%

Food Name	Serv. Size	Total Cal.	Prot. gms	Carbs gms	Sod. mgs	Fiber gms	Fat gms	Chol. mgs	Sat.Fat gms	%Fat Cal.
breast, regular, on sourdough bun ...	1 sandwich	535	37	81	2365	3	10.0	85.0	3	16%
breast, small, on sourdough bun	1 sandwich	363	25	55	1596	2	7.0	58.0	2	16%
Chicken club										
large, on sourdough bun	1 sandwich	1351	88	149	4678	8	45.0	209.0	17	30%
medium on sourdough bun	1 sandwich	686	44	75	2403	4	23.0	106.0	9	30%
small, on sourdough bun	1 sandwich	458	29	50	1591	3	15.0	71.0	6	30%
Corned beef										
large, on sourdough bun	1 sandwich	1134	81	139	4751	6	25.0	167.0	5	20%
regular, on dark rye bun	1 sandwich	587	40	70	2488	4	15.0	84.0	3	23%
small, on dark rye bun	1 sandwich	388	27	47	1625	3	10.0	56.0	2	23%
'Deluxe Original'										
large, on sourdough bun	1 sandwich	2638	143	173	10762	8	152.0	451.0	62	52%
regular, on sourdough bun	1 sandwich	1296	69	87	5405	4	75.0	217.0	29	52%
small, on sourdough bun	1 sandwich	1044	55	60	4275	3	65.0	192.0	26	56%
Dijon chicken										
large, on sourdough bun	1 sandwich	972	74	150	3981	8	10.0	137.0	2	9%
regular, on wheat bun	1 sandwich	497	38	74	2091	6	6.0	68.0	1	11%
small, on wheat bun	1 sandwich	330	25	50	1373	4	4.0	46.0	1	11%
Ham and cheese										
original, large, on sourdough bun ...	1 sandwich	1625	93	163	6807	8	67.0	183.0	29	37%
original, regular, on sourdough bun ...	1 sandwich	789	44	82	3428	4	32.0	83.0	12	36%
original, small, on sourdough bun ...	1 sandwich	537	30	55	2298	3	22.0	58.0	9	37%
'Original'										
large, on sourdough bun	1 sandwich	1917	90	161	6155	8	102.0	246.0	46	48%
regular, on sourdough bun	1 sandwich	941	42	81	3166	4	50.0	122.0	22	48%
small, on sourdough bun	1 sandwich	713	32	55	2327	3	41.0	100.0	17	51%
Pastrami and Swiss										
large, on sourdough bun	1 sandwich	1681	114	148	7211	6	69.0	304.0	32	37%
regular, on dark rye bun	1 sandwich	861	57	74	3718	4	37.0	152.0	17	39%
small, on dark rye bun	1 sandwich	570	38	49	2445	3	24.0	101.0	11	38%
Pesto chicken										
large, on sourdough bun	1 sandwich	999	73	145	3799	7	15.0	141.0	3	13%
regular, on sourdough bun	1 sandwich	512	37	73	1927	4	9.0	71.0	2	16%
small, on sourdough bun	1 sandwich	346	25	49	1297	2	6.0	48.0	1	15%
Philly										
large, on sourdough bun	1 sandwich	1709	121	157	4477	7	66.0	244.0	32	35%
regular, on sourdough bun	1 sandwich	824	57	78	2189	4	32.0	113.0	14	35%
small, on sourdough bun	1 sandwich	559	39	52	1467	2	22.0	78.0	10	35%
Reuben										
corned beef, large, on sourdough bun	1 sandwich	1594	102	147	6944	7	62.0	262.0	25	36%
corned beef, regular, on dark rye bun	1 sandwich	833	51	74	3514	4	35.0	132.0	13	39%
corned beef, small, on dark rye bun	1 sandwich	528	32	50	2269	3	21.0	80.0	7	37%
pastrami, large, on sourdough bun	1 sandwich	1777	113	152	7765	7	77.0	308.0	34	40%
pastrami, regular, on dark rye bun ...	1 sandwich	924	56	77	3924	4	43.0	155.0	18	42%
pastrami, small, on dark rye bun	1 sandwich	619	38	51	2679	3	29.0	103.0	12	42%

Food Name	Serv. Size	Total Cal.	Prot. gms	Carbs gms	Sod. mgs	Fiber gms	Fat gms	Chol. mgs	Sat.Fat gms	%Fat Cal.
turkey, large, on sourdough bun ..... 1 sandwich		1656	101	159	7704	7	69.0	247.0	31	37%
turkey, regular, on dark rye bun ..... 1 sandwich		863	50	80	3893	4	39.0	124.0	16	40%
turkey, small, on dark rye bun ...... 1 sandwich		579	33	54	2659	3	26.0	83.0	11	40%
Roast beef										
large, on sourdough bun .... 1 sandwich		1185	87	145	3362	6	28.0	164.0	6	21%
regular, on sourdough bun .... 1 sandwich		617	43	73	1733	3	17.0	83.0	3	25%
small, on sourdough bun .... 1 sandwich		413	29	49	1162	2	11.0	55.0	2	24%
Roast beef and cheese										
large, on sourdough bun .... 1 sandwich		1749	120	163	4987	8	70.0	255.0	33	36%
regular, on sourdough bun .... 1 sandwich		848	57	82	2451	4	34.0	119.0	14	36%
small, on sourdough bun .... 1 sandwich		580	39	55	1666	3	24.0	83.0	10	36%
Santa Fe chicken										
large, on sourdough bun .... 1 sandwich		1182	82	155	4232	9	29.0	185.0	14	22%
regular, on jalapeño cheese bun .... 1 sandwich		642	43	77	2302	4	19.0	106.0	9	26%
small, on jalapeño cheese bun ..... 1 sandwich		431	29	52	1547	3	13.0	72.0	6	27%
'Texas Schlotzsky's'										
large, on sourdough bun .... 1 sandwich		1544	84	155	6446	6	65.0	184.0	27	38%
regular, on jalapeño cheese bun .... 1 sandwich		816	43	76	3357	3	37.0	98.0	16	41%
small, on jalapeño cheese bun ..... 1 sandwich		561	30	51	2263	2	26.0	69.0	12	42%
Tuna										
albacore, large, on sourdough bun .. 1 sandwich		1000	59	147	3099	6	26.0	122.0	6	22%
albacore, regular, on wheat bun ..... 1 sandwich		533	31	74	1655	4	16.0	69.0	4	26%
albacore, small, on wheat bun ...... 1 sandwich		361	21	50	1122	3	11.0	47.0	3	26%
Tuna melt										
albacore, large, on sourdough bun ... 1 sandwich		1631	93	158	4474	7	77.0	214.0	34	41%
albacore, regular, on wheat bun ..... 1 sandwich		818	45	79	2293	5	40.0	106.0	16	42%
albacore, small, on wheat bun ...... 1 sandwich		562	31	53	1552	3	28.0	74.0	12	43%
Turkey										
breast, smoked, large, on sourdough bun .... 1 sandwich		988	68	150	4229	6	13.0	118.0	2	12%
breast, smoked, regular, on sourdough bun .... 1 sandwich		498	34	75	2123	3	7.0	60.0	1	13%
breast, smoked, small, on sourdough bun .... 1 sandwich		335	23	50	1426	2	5.0	40.0	1	13%
original, large, on sourdough bun ... 1 sandwich		2083	123	166	7535	8	104.0	324.0	45	45%
original, regular, on sourdough bun ... 1 sandwich		1017	58	83	3744	4	51.0	154.0	20	45%
original, small, on sourdough bun ... 1 sandwich		763	43	56	2789	3	41.0	125.0	17	48%
Turkey bacon club										
large, on sourdough bun .... 1 sandwich		1790	108	161	6086	7	80.0	240.0	35	40%
regular, on wheat bun .... 1 sandwich		874	52	79	3009	5	40.0	113.0	15	41%
small, on wheat bun .... 1 sandwich		596	35	53	2012	3	27.0	78.0	11	41%
Turkey guacamole										
large, on sourdough bun .... 1 sandwich		1317	73	166	5255	6	42.0	118.0	6	28%
regular, on sourdough bun .... 1 sandwich		683	36	84	2680	3	24.0	60.0	3	31%
small, on sourdough bun .... 1 sandwich		448	24	56	1764	2	15.0	40.0	2	30%
Vegetable club										
large, on sourdough bun .... 1 sandwich		1112	39	151	2716	9	41.0	46.0	13	33%
regular, on sourdough bun .... 1 sandwich		584	19	76	1435	5	24.0	24.0	7	36%
small, on sourdough bun .... 1 sandwich		393	13	50	962	3	16.0	17.0	5	36%

Food Name	Serv. Size	Total Cal.	Prot. gms	Carbs gms	Sod. mgs	Fiber gms	Fat gms	Chol. mgs	Sat.Fat gms	%Fat Cal.
Vegetarian										
large, on sourdough bun	1 sandwich	966	34	150	2398	8	26.0	48.0	12	24%
regular, on wheat bun	1 sandwich	519	18	75	1329	5	17.0	32.0	7	29%
small, on wheat bun	1 sandwich	351	12	51	889	4	11.0	22.0	5	28%
Western, large, on sourdough bun	1 sandwich	1261	35	150	2235	8	61.0	125.0	28	43%
Western, regular, on sourdough bun	1 sandwich	651	18	75	1161	4	33.0	62.0	14	44%
Western, small, on sourdough bun	1 sandwich	449	12	51	790	3	23.0	47.0	10	45%
SIDE DISH										
coleslaw, country style	5 oz	225	1	16	288	1	16.0	5.0	3	68%
coleslaw, shredded	5 oz	225	1	16	388	1	16.0	19.0	3	68%
macaroni salad	5 oz	338	4	23	619	1	23.0	9.0	4	66%
potato salad, 'Choice'	5 oz	253	2	18	525	1	18.0	9.0	3	67%
potato salad, diced, w/egg	5 oz	216	3	18	600	1	13.0	38.0	2	58%
potato salad, mustard/egg	5 oz	225	2	17	534	1	15.0	5.0	2	64%
seven bean medley	8-oz cup	145	7	24	1260	8	2.0	0.0	1	13%
SOUP										
Boston clam chowder	8-oz cup	233	5	24	1062	1	15.0	10.0	1	54%
broccoli cheese	8-oz cup	252	7	23	1104	1	17.0	17.0	4	56%
broccoli, cream of	8-oz cup	206	4	25	1152	1	13.0	15.0	3	50%
cauliflower cheese	8-oz cup	252	3	24	993	1	19.0	11.0	4	61%
chicken gumbo	8-oz cup	110	4	13	1114	2	5.0	20.0	1	40%
chicken noodle, old-fashioned	8-oz cup	122	8	18	1104	1	2.0	39.0	1	15%
chicken tortilla	8-oz cup	167	10	24	1026	3	3.0	22.0	1	17%
chicken, w/wild rice	8-oz cup	378	10	24	1201	1	28.0	78.0	12	65%
corn chowder	8-oz cup	284	2	38	1010	1	17.0	6.0	3	49%
creamy turkey vegetable	8-oz cup	218	7	21	871	1	14.0	22.0	2	53%
French onion	8-oz cup	78	3	9	1716	0	3.0	0.0	1	36%
minestrone	8-oz cup	89	3	17	1048	3	1.0	0.0	0	10%
potato, cream of, w/bacon	8-oz cup	226	2	31	1209	2	13.0	5.0	1	47%
ravioli tomato	8-oz cup	111	6	21	1115	1	2.0	17.0	0	14%
red beans and rice	8-oz cup	167	8	32	934	4	1.0	0.0	0	5%
tomato Florentine	8-oz cup	100	3	19	1182	1	1.0	0.0	0	9%
vegetable beef barley	8-oz cup	100	6	12	1160	2	3.0	11.0	1	27%
vegetable cheese	8-oz cup	289	6	24	1338	2	19.0	28.0	6	59%
vegetable, lumberjack	8-oz cup	133	3	19	1482	6	6.0	6.0	2	38%
vegetable, vegetarian	8-oz cup	138	3	20	1536	6	6.0	6.0	2	37%
Wisconsin cheese	8-oz cup	319	4	26	1104	1	25.0	22.0	7	65%
SHAKEY'S PIZZA										
CHICKEN ENTRÉE										
fried, w/potatoes	3 pieces	947	57	51	2293	0	56.0	0.0	0	54%
fried, w/potatoes	5 pieces	1700	97	130	5327	0	90.0	0.0	0	47%
PIZZA										
Cheese										
homestyle pan crust, 12-inch pie	1/10 pie	303	14	31	591	0	13.7	21.0	0	41%
thick crust, regular, 12-inch pie	1/10 pie	170	9	22	421	0	4.8	13.0	0	26%

Food Name	Serv. Size	Total Cal.	Prot. gms	Carbs gms	Sod. mgs	Fiber gms	Fat gms	Chol. mgs	Sat.Fat gms	%Fat Cal.
thick crust, 'Shakey's Special'										
12-inch pie	1/10 pie	208	13	22	423	0	8.3	18.0	0	35%
thin crust, 'Shakey's Special'										
12-inch pie	1/10 pie	171	13	14	475	0	8.7	16.0	0	42%
thin crust, regular, 12-inch pie	1/10 pie	133	8	13	323	0	5.2	14.0	0	35%
Ham and cheese, 'Hot Ham and										
Cheese'	1 serving	550	36	56	2135	0	21.0	0.0	0	34%
Pepperoni										
homestyle pan crust 12-inch pie	1/10 pie	343	16	31	740	0	15.4	27.0	0	42%
thick crust, 12-inch pie	1/10 pie	185	10	22	422	0	6.4	17.0	0	31%
thin crust, 12-inch pie	1/10 pie	148	8	13	403	0	6.9	14.0	0	42%
Sausage and mushroom										
homestyle pan crust, 12-inch pie	1/10 pie	343	16	31	677	0	16.9	24.0	0	44%
thick crust, 12-inch pie	1/10 pie	179	10	22	420	0	5.6	15.0	0	28%
thin crust, 12-inch pie	1/10 pie	141	9	13	336	0	6.0	13.0	0	38%
Sausage and pepperoni										
homestyle pan crust, 12-inch pie	1/10 pie	374	17	31	676	0	19.9	24.0	0	48%
thick crust, 12-inch pie	1/10 pie	177	11	22	424	0	8.0	19.0	0	35%
thin crust, 12-inch pie	1/10 pie	166	9	13	397	0	8.4	17.0	0	46%
'Sausage Supreme'										
homestyle pan crust, vegetable,										
12-inch pie	1/10 pie	320	15	32	652	0	14.7	21.0	0	41%
'Special' homestyle pan crust,										
12-inch pie	1/10 pie	384	18	32	878	0	20.7	29.0	0	48%
'Thai Chicken' thick crust, 12-inch pie	1/10 pie	162	9	22	418	0	4.1	13.0	0	23%
POTATO, wedges	15 pieces	950	17	120	3703	0	36.0	0.0	0	37%
SANDWICH										
'Hot Ham and Cheese'	1 sandwich	550	36	56	2135	0	21.0	0.0	0	34%
'Super Hot Hero'	1 sandwich	810	36	67	2688	0	44.0	0.0	0	49%
SPAGHETTI ENTRÉE, w/meat sauce										
and garlic bread	1 serving	940	26	134	1904	0	33.0	0.0	0	32%
SHONEY'S										
BISCUIT	1 serving	170	3	22	364	0	8.1	0.0	0	43%
BREAD, Grecian	1 serving	80	2	13	94	0	2.2	0.0	0	25%
BREAKFAST										
bacon	3 strips	109	6	0	303	0	9.4	16.0	0	78%
croissant, plain	1 serving	260	5	22	260	0	16.0	2.0	0	57%
egg, fried	1 egg	159	6	1	69	0	14.7	274.0	0	83%
ham	2 slices	59	7	1	526	0	2.1	28.0	0	38%
honey bun	1 bun	265	4	32	33	0	14.0	3.0	0	47%
pancake, 6-inch	1 cake	91	2	20	522	0	0.2	0.0	0	2%
sausage	1 patty	103	4	0	161	0	9.6	17.0	0	85%
syrup, low calorie	2.2 oz	98	0	24	0	0	0.0	0.0	0	0%
toast, w/butter	2 slices	163	4	25	296	1	5.2	0.0	0	29%
CHEESEBURGER, 'Mushroom/Swiss										
Burger'	1 burger	616	32	29	1135	1	41.7	106.0	0	61%
CHICKEN ENTRÉE										
charbroiled, 'LightSide'	1 serving	239	39	1	592	0	7.0	85.0	0	28%
tenders, 'America's Favorites'	1 serving	388	35	17	239	0	20.4	64.0	0	47%
COMBINATION ENTRÉE										
'Fish N' Shrimp'	1 serving	487	28	37	644	0	25.5	127.0	0	47%

Food Name	Serv. Size	Total Cal.	Prot. gms	Carbs gms	Sod. mgs	Fiber gms	Fat gms	Chol. mgs	Sat.Fat gms	%Fat Cal.
'Italian Feast'	1 serving	500	38	44	369	1	19.6	74.0	0	35%
ribeye steak and chicken, charbroiled	1 serving	605	35	0	211	0	50.5	141.0	0	76%
sirloin and chicken, charbroiled	1 serving	357	32	0	160	0	24.5	99.0	0	63%
steak and chicken, charbroiled	8-oz serving	435	31	0	280	0	34.4	123.0	0	71%
'Steak N' Shrimp' charbroiled shrimp	1 serving	361	37	1	198	0	22.6	141.0	0	58%
'Steak N' Shrimp' fried shrimp	1 serving	507	37	15	249	0	32.7	150.0	0	59%
CONDIMENTS. See also Salad dressing.										
gravy, country	3 oz	114	1	6	358	0	9.8	2.0	0	76%
onion, sautéed	2.5-oz serving	37	1	4	221	1	2.1	0.0	0	48%
sweet and sour sauce, souffle cup	1 cup	58	0	15	5	0	0.0	0.0	0	0%
tartar sauce, souffle cup	1 cup	84	0	4	177	0	7.7	11.0	0	82%
DESSERT										
apple pie, à la mode	1 serving	492	6	67	574	0	23.0	35.0	0	41%
brownie, walnut, à la mode	1 serving	576	10	61	435	0	33.7	35.0	0	52%
carrot cake	1 serving	500	9	56	476	0	26.0	37.0	0	47%
hot fudge cake	1 serving	522	7	82	485	0	19.7	27.0	0	33%
hot fudge sundae	1 serving	451	7	60	226	0	22.0	60.0	0	42%
strawberry pie	1 serving	332	2	45	247	2	16.7	0.0	0	45%
strawberry sundae	1 serving	380	6	48	145	0	19.0	69.0	0	44%
FISH										
baked, 'LightSide'	1 serving	170	35	2	1641	0	1.0	83.0	0	6%
fried, 'Light'	1 serving	297	20	22	536	0	14.4	65.0	0	44%
FISH ENTRÉE, fried, w/fries	1 serving	639	32	50	873	3	34.8	103.0	0	49%
HAMBURGER										
'All-American'	1 burger	501	25	27	597	1	32.6	86.0	0	59%
'Old Fashioned'	1 burger	470	25	26	681	1	28.2	82.0	0	56%
'Shoney Burger'	1 burger	498	23	22	782	0	35.7	79.0	0	64%
w/bacon	1 burger	591	29	29	801	1	40.0	86.0	0	61%
HAMBURGER PATTY, beef, light	1 serving	289	21	0	187	0	22.9	82.0	0	71%
LASAGNA ENTRÉE										
'America's Favorites'	1 serving	297	8	45	870	3	9.8	26.0	0	29%
light, 'LightSide'	1 serving	297	8	45	870	0	10.0	26.0	0	30%
LIVER ENTRÉE, w/onions, 'America's Favorites'	1 serving	411	35	15	321	1	22.9	529.0	0	51%
SALAD DRESSING										
Biscayne, low-calorie	2 tbsp	62	6	1	334	0	1.0	0.0	0	24%
blue cheese	2 tbsp	113	0	0	109	0	13.0	15.0	0	100%
French	2 tbsp	124	2	2	204	0	12.0	12.0	0	87%
French rue	2 tbsp	122	5	2	364	0	10.0	0.0	0	76%
honey mustard	2 tbsp	165	2	2	5	0	17.0	18.0	0	89%
Italian, creamy	2 tbsp	135	0	1	454	0	15.0	0.0	0	97%
Italian, golden	2 tbsp	141	0	1	302	0	15.0	0.0	0	97%
Italian, nonfat	2 tbsp	10	0	2	615	0	0.0	0.0	0	0%
Ranch	2 tbsp	95	0	0	10	0	10.0	15.0	0	100%
Thousand Island	2 tbsp	130	1	2	179	0	13.0	12.0	0	91%
SANDWICH										
cheese and bacon, grilled	1 sandwich	440	18	28	1200	1	28.2	36.0	0	58%
cheese, grilled	1 sandwich	454	17	29	1519	0	29.0	0.0	0	59%

Food Name	Serv. Size	Total Cal.	Prot. gms	Carbs gms	Sod. mgs	Fiber gms	Fat gms	Chol. mgs	Sat.Fat gms	%Fat Cal.
chicken, charbroiled	1 sandwich	451	43	28	1002	1	17.0	90.0	0	35%
chicken fillet	1 sandwich	464	30	39	585	1	21.2	51.0	0	41%
fish	1 sandwich	323	12	41	740	0	12.7	21.0	0	35%
ham club, on whole wheat	1 sandwich	642	37	45	2105	11	35.5	78.0	0	49%
ham, baked	1 sandwich	290	19	28	1263	2	10.3	42.0	0	33%
patty melt	1 sandwich	640	39	30	826	7	41.7	121.0	0	58%
Philly steak	1 sandwich	673	32	37	1242	0	44.0	103.0	0	59%
Reuben	1 sandwich	596	33	32	3873	6	34.7	138.0	0	55%
'Slim Jim'	1 sandwich	484	27	40	1620	1	23.9	57.0	0	44%
steak, country fried	1 sandwich	588	25	67	1501	1	25.8	29.0	0	39%
turkey club, on whole wheat	1 sandwich	635	44	44	1289	10	32.7	100.0	0	46%
SEAFOOD PLATTER ENTRÉE	1 serving	566	33	46	893	0	28.0	127.0	0	45%
SHRIMP										
bite-sized	1 serving	387	16	25	1266	0	24.7	140.0	0	57%
charbroiled	1 serving	138	25	3	170	0	3.0	162.0	0	20%
SHRIMP ENTRÉE										
boiled	1 serving	93	20	0	210	0	1.0	182.0	0	10%
sampler	1 serving	412	26	26	783	0	22.7	217.0	0	50%
'Shrimper's Feast' regular	1 serving	383	17	30	216	0	22.2	125.0	0	52%
'Shrimper's Feast' large	1 serving	575	25	45	324	0	33.3	188.0	0	52%
SIDE DISH										
ambrosia salad	1/4 cup	75	1	12	167	1	3.3	0.0	0	38%
apple grape surprise salad	1/4 cup	19	0	5	2	0	0.0	0.0	0	0%
baked potato	10-oz serving	264	6	61	16	7	0.3	0.0	0	1%
beet-onion salad	1/4 cup	25	1	3	167	1	1.3	0.0	0	45%
broccoli-cauliflower-ranch salad	1/4 cup	65	1	2	12	1	6.4	9.0	0	85%
carrot-apple salad	1/4 cup	99	1	4	10	1	9.1	8.0	0	81%
coleslaw	1/4 cup	69	1	5	106	1	5.1	7.0	0	65%
cucumber salad, lite	1/4 cup	12	0	3	344	0	0.1	0.0	0	7%
'Don's Pasta Salad'	1/4 cup	82	2	9	223	0	4.6	0.0	0	50%
french fries	3-oz serving	189	3	29	273	3	7.5	0.0	0	35%
french fries	4-oz serving	252	4	39	364	4	9.9	0.0	0	34%
'Fruit Delight Salad'	1/4 cup	54	1	10	2	1	1.6	0.0	0	25%
grits	3 oz	57	1	6	62	0	3.2	0.0	0	51%
grits, instant	100 grams	67	1	7	73	0	3.8	0.0	0	51%
hash browns	3 oz	90	2	14	50	0	3.1	0.0	0	31%
home fries	3 oz	115	2	19	53	0	3.7	0.0	0	29%
Italian vegetable salad	1/4 cup	11	0	3	110	1	0.1	0.0	0	7%
kidney bean salad	1/4 cup	55	3	7	154	2	2.1	2.0	0	33%
macaroni salad	1/4 cup	207	4	17	382	0	13.9	14.0	0	60%
mixed squash salad	1/4 cup	49	1	2	230	0	4.1	0.0	0	73%
mushroom, sauteed	3-oz serving	75	2	4	968	1	6.5	0.0	0	71%
onion rings	1 ring	52	1	5	102	0	3.1	2.0	0	54%
Oriental salad	1/4 cup	79	1	13	31	1	2.7	1.0	0	30%
pea salad	1/4 cup	73	3	4	89	2	5.5	42.0	0	67%
rice	3.5-oz serving	137	2	23	765	0	3.7	1.0	0	25%
rotelli pasta	1/4 cup	78	1	9	82	0	4.0	0.0	0	47%
seigan salad	1/4 cup	72	2	8	122	1	3.6	5.0	0	44%
snow salad	1/4 cup	72	1	9	18	0	4.1	0.0	0	49%
spaghetti salad	1/4 cup	81	2	9	20	0	4.6	0.0	0	50%

Food Name	Serv. Size	Total Cal.	Prot. gms	Carbs gms	Sod. mgs	Fiber gms	Fat gms	Chol. mgs	Sat.Fat gms	%Fat Cal.
spring salad	1/4 cup	38	1	2	162	1	2.9	0.0	0	67%
summer salad	1/4 cup	114	1	2	233	1	11.6	0.0	0	89%
three-bean salad	1/4 cup	96	1	12	189	1	5.1	0.0	0	46%
Waldorf salad	1/4 cup	81	1	9	68	1	5.2	2.0	0	55%
SOUP										
bean	6 oz	63	4	10	479	1	1.1	4.0	0	15%
beef, w/cabbage	6 oz	86	6	9	503	2	3.0	13.0	0	30%
broccoli, cream of	6 oz	75	2	11	415	0	4.6	1.0	0	46%
cauliflower	6 oz	124	4	12	560	1	9.2	12.0	0	57%
Cheddar chowder	6 oz	91	3	14	948	0	2.3	0.0	0	23%
cheese Florentine, w/ham	6 oz	110	4	12	890	1	7.8	11.0	0	53%
chicken, cream of	6 oz	136	5	14	1164	0	8.9	11.0	0	53%
chicken gumbo	6 oz	60	4	7	1050	0	2.0	0.0	0	29%
chicken noodle	6 oz	62	3	9	127	0	1.4	14.0	0	20%
chicken vegetable, cream of	6 oz	79	4	13	714	0	1.3	0.0	0	15%
chicken w/rice	6 oz	72	3	13	117	1	0.5	6.0	0	6%
clam chowder	6 oz	94	2	10	66	0	5.4	0.0	0	52%
corn chowder	6 oz	148	4	22	510	0	4.7	0.0	0	29%
onion	6 oz	29	1	2	88	0	2.0	1.0	0	63%
potato	6 oz	102	1	17	335	2	3.4	0.0	0	30%
tomato, w/vegetable	6 oz	46	2	10	314	0	0.3	0.0	0	5%
tomato Florentine	6 oz	63	2	11	683	0	1.1	0.0	0	16%
vegetable beef	6 oz	82	4	14	1254	0	1.5	5.0	0	16%
SPAGHETTI ENTRÉE										
'America's Favorites'	1 serving	496	24	63	387	2	16.3	55.0	0	30%
SPAGHETTI ENTRÉE, LIGHT										
light, 'LightSide'	1 serving	248	12	32	194	0	8.0	28.0	0	29%
STEAK, sirloin, charbroiled	6 oz	357	32	0	160	0	24.5	99.0	0	63%
STEAK ENTRÉE, country fried steak										
'America's Favorites'	1 serving	449	19	34	1177	1	27.2	27.0	0	53%
SIZZLER										
BEEF										
roast beef, sliced	2/3 oz	17	3	0	276	0	0.3	8.0	0	16%
steak, New York strip	12 oz	600	70	5	200	0	35.0	180.0	0	51%
steak, sirloin	6.25 oz	447	55	0	245	0	34.0	120.0	12	58%
BEEF PATTY	8 oz	530	42	0	150	0	38.0	156.0	15	67%
BREAD, focaccia	2 pieces	108	2	9	134	0	7.0	1.0	1	59%
BREADSTICK, garlic, soft	1 oz	75	2	15	112	0	0.5	0.0	0	6%
CHICKEN										
breast, lemon herb	5 oz	151	27	27	0	0	4.0	0.0	0	14%
wing	1 oz	73	4	4	136	0	4.0	20.0	1	53%
wing, Cajun	3 oz	201	16	2	435	0	14.4	111.0	0	65%
wing, Southern	1 oz	73	5	4	135	0	6.0	20.0	1	62%
wing, whole, Southern	1 oz	74	4	4	285	0	4.8	18.0	2	59%
CHICKEN ENTRÉE, w/noodles	6 oz	164	13	20	524	0	4.0	40.0	1	21%
CHICKEN PATTY, 'Malibu'	1 patty	368	27	12	0	0	25.0	0.0	0	59%
CHILI, 'Grande' w/beans	6 oz	100	5	18	1190	0	1.0	0.0	0	9%
CONDIMENTS										
buttery dipping sauce	1.5 oz	330	0	0	0	0	37.0	0.0	7	100%
guacamole	1 oz	42	0	2	425	0	4.0	0.0	1	82%

Food Name	Serv. Size	Total Cal.	Prot. gms	Carbs gms	Sod. mgs	Fiber gms	Fat gms	Chol. mgs	Sat.Fat gms	%Fat Cal.
guacamole, extra chunky	3.5 oz serving	285	3	7	0	0	18.4	0.0	0	80%
hibachi sauce	1.5 oz	57	0	11	707	0	0.0	0.0	0	0%
Malibu sauce	1.5 oz	283	0	0	354	0	31.0	28.0	6	100%
margarine, whipped	1.5 tbsp	105	0	0	146	0	12.0	0.0	2	100%
marinade	1 oz	13	0	3	90	0	0.0	0.0	0	0%
nacho cheese sauce	2 oz	120	5	3	600	0	10.0	30.0	5	74%
pepper, bell, salad bar item	2 oz	8	1	2	1	1	0.0	0.0	0	0%
salsa	1 oz	7	0	2	156	0	0.0	0.0	0	0%
tartar sauce	1.5 oz	170	0	6	453	0	17.0	14.0	3	86%
turkey ham, salad bar item	1 oz	62	4	0	376	0	5.0	19.0	2	74%
CORNED BEEF, sliced	1 oz	45	8	0	55	0	1.5	0.0	0	30%
CRAB, snow, legs and claws,	3.5 oz	91	21	0	539	0	1.1	55.0	0	11%
CRAB, IMITATION, shredded	3.5 oz serving	104	12	14	864	0	1.0	22.0	0	8%
CROISSANT, mini	1 croissant	120	2	12	95	0	8.0	4.0	3	56%
DESSERT										
'Parfait Salad'	3.5 oz serving	84	2	17	66	0	1.7	0.0	2	18%
yogurt, frozen, chocolate, soft-serve	4 oz	136	1	24	100	0	4.0	0.0	4	26%
yogurt, frozen, vanilla, soft-serve	4 oz	136	1	24	100	0	4.0	0.0	4	26%
DESSERT TOPPING										
chocolate syrup	1 oz	90	0	21	15	0	0.0	0.0	0	0%
strawberry, nonfat	1 oz	70	0	18	5	0	0.0	0.0	0	0%
whipped	1 tbsp	12	0	1	0	0	1.0	0.0	1	69%
FISH NUGGETS	1 oz	40	4	5	100	0	0.0	10.0	0	0%
HALIBUT, steak	6 oz	180	36	0	103	0	2.0	86.0	1	11%
HAMBURGER, w/lettuce and tomato	1 serving	626	45	36	335	1	33.0	142.0	12	48%
LASAGNA										
w/meat	8 oz	327	21	23	657	0	13.0	37.0	6	40%
vegetable	8 oz	245	15	29	553	0	8.0	19.0	5	29%
MACARONI AND CHEESE	6 oz	214	10	22	590	0	9.0	26.0	5	39%
MEATBALL	4 meatballs	157	9	5	461	1	11.0	30.0	5	64%
PASTA										
fettuccine	2 oz	80	3	15	5	0	1.0	5.0	0	11%
fettuccine, whole egg, dry	2 oz	210	9	40	8	0	1.0	0.0	1	4%
ravioli, cheese	4 oz	260	10	47	270	0	4.0	20.0	2	14%
spaghetti	2 oz	80	3	16	1	1	0.0	0.0	0	0%
POLLACK, breaded	4 oz	140	14	18	280	0	1.0	35.0	0	7%
SALAD DRESSING										
bacon, hot	1 tbsp	40	0	58	90	0	20.0	0.0	0	44%
blue cheese	1 oz	111	1	1	168	0	12.0	8.0	4	93%
honey mustard	1 oz	160	0	4	110	0	16.0	10.0	2	90%
Italian, lite	1 oz	14	0	2	350	0	0.0	0.0	0	0%
Italian, Parmesan	1 oz	100	0	2	450	0	10.0	0.0	2	92%
Japanese rice vinegar, nonfat	1 oz	10	0	2	172	0	0.0	0.0	0	0%
Malibu	1 tbsp	100	0	0	125	0	11.0	10.0	2	100%
ranch	1 oz	120	0	2	240	0	12.0	10.0	2	93%
ranch, lower calorie	1 oz	90	0	4	270	0	8.0	10.0	2	82%
sour	1.5 oz	89	0	0	44	0	9.0	0.0	8	100%
sour	2 tbsp	60	0	0	30	0	6.0	0.0	5	100%
Thousand Island	1 oz	143	0	3	125	0	15.0	11.0	2	92%

Food Name	Serv. Size	Total Cal.	Prot. gms	Carbs gms	Sod. mgs	Fiber gms	Fat gms	Chol. mgs	Sat.Fat gms	%Fat Cal.
SALMON	8 oz	247	32	0	232	0	12.0	41.0	2	46%
SCALLOP, breaded, approx 30–40	4 oz	160	14	24	393	0	1.0	18.0	0	6%
SHRIMP										
broiled	5 oz	150	23	0	377	0	6.0	218.0	1	37%
butterfly, breaded, approx 16–20	3.5 oz	220	10	16	440	0	13.0	50.0	0	53%
butterfly, breaded, approx 10–12	3.5 oz	145	10	14	280	0	0.1	0.0	0	1%
butterfly, Cajun, breaded, approx 16–20	3.5 oz	145	10	24	280	0	0.1	0.0	0	1%
butterfly, lemon pepper, breaded, approx 21–25	2 oz	190	5	38	211	0	1.0	5.0	0	5%
Cajun, breaded, approx 80–90	3.5 oz	140	10	22	198	0	0.9	0.0	0	6%
mini, breaded, approx 50–60	3.5 oz	140	10	22	198	0	0.9	0.0	0	6%
mini, Cajun, breaded, approx 40–50	3.5 oz	141	10	22	200	0	0.9	0.0	0	6%
scampi	5 oz	143	27	0	386	0	3.0	150.0	1	20%
tempura-battered, approx 21–25	3 oz	155	10	13	442	0	8.0	74.0	3	44%
SIDE DISH										
avocado, salad bar item	1/2 avocado	153	2	6	11	3	15.0	0.0	2	81%
baked potato, flesh only	4 oz	105	2	24	6	2	0.0	0.0	0	0%
broccoli, salad bar item	1/2 cup	12	1	2	12	1	0.0	0.0	0	0%
carrot-raisin salad	2 oz	130	1	10	104	1	10.0	10.0	2	67%
cauliflower, battered, not fried	3.5 oz serving	184	3	21	49	0	10.3	1.0	0	49%
cheese toast	1 piece	273	6	16	494	1	21.0	5.0	5	68%
Chinese chicken salad	2 oz	54	4	6	119	1	2.0	10.0	0	31%
corn nuggets	3 oz	117	3	22	325	0	8.4	0.0	0	44%
cottage cheese, low-fat	1/2 cup	100	14	4	390	0	2.0	8.0	1	20%
french fries	4 oz	358	5	45	245	4	12.0	0.0	6	35%
four-bean salad	3.5 oz serving	104	3	19	226	0	2.5	0.0	0	21%
grapes, salad bar item	1/2 cup	29	0	8	1	1	0.0	0.0	0	0%
jicama, salad bar item	2 oz	13	1	3	1	0	0.0	0.0	0	0%
jicama salad, spicy	2 oz	16	0	4	28	0	0.0	0.0	0	0%
kidney beans, salad bar item	1/4 cup	52	3	10	222	4	0.0	0.0	0	0%
kiwifruit, salad bar item	2 oz	35	1	8	3	2	0.0	0.0	0	0%
lettuce, Romaine, salad bar item	1 cup	9	1	1	4	1	0.0	0.0	0	0%
macaroni and cheddar salad	3.5 oz serving	185	3	16	476	0	12.5	14.0	4	60%
Mediterranean Minted fruit salad	2 oz	29	1	7	11	0	0.0	0.0	0	0%
'Mexican Fiesta Salad'	2 oz	54	2	10	99	1	1.0	0.0	0	16%
okra, breaded, not fried	3.5 oz serving	105	3	24	503	0	0.5	1.0	0	4%
onion rings, steak cut, breaded, not fried	.5 oz serving	395	5	39	558	0	24.4	0.0	0	56%
'Oriental Pasta Salad'	3.5 oz serving	114	4	23	781	0	1.6	1.0	0	12%
potato and egg salad	3.5 oz serving	140	2	16	340	0	7.8	28.0	1	50%
potato salad, 'Old Fashioned'	2 oz	84	1	10	231	1	5.0	8.0	1	51%
potato salad, 'Old Fashioned'	3.5 oz serving	150	2	17	416	0	8.7	23.0	1	51%
potato salad, red, herb	2 oz	121	1	9	271	1	9.0	9.0	1	67%
potato salad, red, herb	3.5 oz serving	213	2	15	437	0	16.2	15.0	2	68%
potato skin	2 oz	160	2	22	463	3	8.0	0.0	1	43%
refried beans	3 oz	120	5	16	320	0	4.0	2.0	2	30%
rice pilaf	6 oz	256	4	47	866	1	5.0	0.0	1	18%

Food Name	Serv. Size	Total Cal.	Prot. gms	Carbs gms	Sod. mgs	Fiber gms	Fat gms	Chol. mgs	Sat.Fat gms	%Fat Cal.
'Seafood Louis' pasta salad	2 oz	64	3	9	139	1	2.0	17.0	0	27%
seafood salad	2 oz	56	3	4	255	0	3.0	7.0	1	49%
shell pasta salad	3.5 oz serving	112	3	19	591	0	2.7	1.0	1	21%
spinach, salad bar item	1/2 cup	6	1	1	22	1	0.0	0.0	0	0%
teriyaki beef salad	2 oz	49	4	5	136	1	2.0	7.0	1	33%
tuna pasta salad	2 oz	133	6	6	188	0	10.0	10.0	1	65%
tuna salad	3.5 oz serving	353	8	7	296	0	32.9	44.0	5	83%
SOUP										
broccoli cheese soup	4 oz	139	3	10	355	0	9.0	8.0	2	61%
chicken w/noodle	4 oz	31	2	4	495	0	1.0	7.0	0	27%
clam chowder	4 oz	118	3	11	511	0	6.0	6.0	0	49%
minestrone, nonfat	4 oz	36	1	7	443	2	0.0	1.0	0	0%
vegetable, vegetarian	6 oz	50	2	6	630	0	1.0	0.0	0	22%
vegetable sirloin soup	4 oz	60	6	6	364	0	2.0	10.0	1	27%
SWORDFISH	8 oz	315	45	0	331	0	14.0	89.0	3	41%
TACO SHELL	1 shell	50	1	7	20	1	2.0	0.0	0	36%
TUNA, yellowfin	3.5 oz serving	125	15	0	50	0	4.0	65.0	1	38%

SKIPPER'S

Food Name	Serv. Size	Total Cal.	Prot. gms	Carbs gms	Sod. mgs	Fiber gms	Fat gms	Chol. mgs	Sat.Fat gms	%Fat Cal.
CHICKEN ENTRÉE										
'Lite Catch' 3 pieces, w/small green salad	1 serving	305	26	17	673	0	15.0	58.0	0	44%
tenderloin strips, 5 pieces, w/fries	1 serving	793	44	69	798	0	38.0	77.0	0	43%
CHICKEN STRIPS, 'Create A Catch'	1 serving	82	8	4	150	0	4.0	15.0	0	43%
CLAM ENTRÉE, 'Basket' strips w/fries	1 serving	1003	22	90	569	0	70.0	14.0	0	58%
COD ENTRÉE										
3 pieces, thick cut, w/fries	1 serving	665	27	68	1054	0	32.0	38.0	0	43%
4 pieces, thick cut w/fries	1 serving	759	34	74	1388	0	36.0	50.0	0	43%
5 pieces, thick cut, w/fries	1 serving	853	42	80	1723	0	41.0	62.0	0	43%
COMBINATION ENTRÉE										
'Combos' clam strips, 1 piece fish, fries	1 serving	868	25	81	667	0	54.0	61.0	0	53%
'Combos' jumbo shrimp, 1 piece fish, fries	1 serving	720	24	75	1268	0	36.0	91.0	0	45%
'Combos' original shrimp, 1 piece fish, fries	1 serving	728	24	77	943	0	37.0	105.0	0	45%
'Combos' oysters, 1 piece fish, fries	1 serving	885	25	95	809	0	44.0	80.0	0	45%
'Lite Catch' 1 piece fish, 2 pieces chicken, small green salad	1 serving	399	29	24	880	0	21.0	96.0	0	47%
3-piece, chicken strip, fish, fries	1 serving	805	80	72	858	0	40.0	100.0	0	37%
3-piece, chicken strip, shrimp, fries	1 serving	800	36	77	1036	0	39.0	97.0	0	44%
DESSERT										
gelatin, nonfat, 'Jell-O' 'Create A Catch'	1 serving	55	1	12	35	0	0.0	0.0	0	0%
root beer float	1 serving	302	3	33	66	0	10.0	10.0	0	38%
FISH										
fillet, 'Create A Catch'	1 serving	175	11	11	357	0	10.0	53.0	0	51%
FISH ENTRÉE										
1 fish fillet, w/fries	1 serving	558	17	51	408	0	28.0	55.0	0	48%
2 fish fillets, w/fries	1 serving	733	28	71	765	0	38.0	108.0	0	46%

Food Name	Serv. Size	Total Cal.	Prot. gms	Carbs gms	Sod. mgs	Fiber gms	Fat gms	Chol. mgs	Sat.Fat gms	%Fat Cal.
3 fish fillets, w/fries	1 serving	908	39	82	1122	0	48.0	160.0	0	47%
'Lite Catch' 2 pieces, w/small green salad	1 serving	409	25	27	937	0	23.0	119.0	0	50%
FISH SANDWICH										
'Create A Catch'	1 sandwich	524	19	43	1191	0	33.0	86.0	0	55%
'Create A Catch' double	1 sandwich	698	30	54	1548	0	73.0	139.0	0	66%
SIDE DISH										
baked potato	1 serving	145	4	32	6	0	0.0	0.0	0	0%
coleslaw.....................	.5 oz serving	289	2	10	329	0	27.0	50.0	0	84%
french fries, 'Create A Catch'	1 serving	383	6	50	51	0	18.0	2.0	0	42%
Soup										
clam chowder, 'Create A Catch' cup ...	1 serving	100	3	14	525	0	3.5	12.0	0	32%
clam chowder, 'Create A Catch' pint ...	1 serving	200	5	19	1050	0	7.0	24.0	0	40%
salmon chowder, 'Alder Smoked Salmon' .....'.....................	6 oz	166	13	14	73	0	7.0	0.0	0	37%
OYSTER ENTRÉE, w/fries 'Basket'	1 serving	1038	28	118	853	0	51.0	52.0	0	44%
SALAD										
green, small, 'Lite Catch'	1 salad	59	3	6	223	0	3.0	13.0	0	43%
shrimp and seafood	1 salad	167	23	15	657	0	3.0	80.0	0	15%
side	1 salad	24	0	4	8	0	0.0	0.0	0	0%
SALAD DRESSING										
salad dressing, blue cheese, premium ..	1 pouch	222	1	4	240	0	23.0	8.0	0	91%
salad dressing, Italian, gourmet	1 pouch	140	0	2	200	0	15.0	0.0	0	94%
salad dressing, Italian, low-calorie	1 pouch	17	0	2	680	0	1.0	0.0	0	53%
salad dressing, ranch house	1 pouch	188	1	2	302	0	20.0	0.0	0	94%
salad dressing, Thousand Island	1 pouch	160	0	8	415	0	14.0	6.0	0	80%
tartar sauce	1 tbsp	65	0	0	102	0	7.0	4.0	0	100%
SALMON, baked	4.4 oz	270	39	1	504	0	11.0	70.0	0	38%
SEAFOOD ENTRÉE, w/fries 'Skipper's Platter Basket'	1 serving	1038	32	97	1202	0	63.0	111.0	0	52%
SHRIMP ENTRÉE										
w/fries, 'Basket'	1 serving	723	20	82	1121	0	36.0	102.0	0	44%
w/fries, jumbo, 'Basket'	1 serving	707	20	79	911	0	35.0	73.0	0	44%
w/seafood salad, 'Lite Catch'	1 serving	167	23	15	657	0	3.0	80.0	0	15%

SONIC
CHEESEBURGER

Food Name	Serv. Size	Total Cal.	Prot. gms	Carbs gms	Sod. mgs	Fiber gms	Fat gms	Chol. mgs	Sat.Fat gms	%Fat Cal.
#1	1 serving	70	4	0	267	0	5.8	18.0	0	75%
#2	1 serving	70	4	0	267	0	5.8	18.0	0	74%
jalapeño, double meat and cheese	1 serving	638	44	22	1358	0	40.6	136.0	0	58%
mini	1 serving	281	17	20	644	0	14.4	45.0	0	47%
w/bacon	1 serving	548	28	23	839	0	38.6	87.0	0	63%
CHILI PIE	1 serving	327	12	20	313	0	22.6	28.0	0	62%
CORN DOG	1 sandwich	280	7	30	700	0	15.0	35.0	0	48%
HAMBURGER										
#1	1 serving	409	20	23	444	0	26.6	58.0	0	58%
#2	1 serving	323	20	23	549	0	15.7	50.0	0	45%
hickory	1 serving	314	20	23	459	0	15.7	50.0	0	45%
mini	1 serving	246	14	20	510	0	11.5	36.0	0	43%

Food Name	Serv. Size	Total Cal.	Prot. gms	Carbs gms	Sod. mgs	Fiber gms	Fat gms	Chol. mgs	Sat.Fat gms	%Fat Cal.
'Super Sonic' double meat and cheese, w/mayo	1 serving	730	44	24	1023	0	51.5	144.0	0	63%
'Super Sonic' double meat and cheese, w/mustard	1 serving	644	44	24	1128	0	40.7	136.0	0	57%
HOT DOG										
'Cheese Coney' extra long	1 serving	635	24	45	632	0	39.0	65.0	0	56%
'Cheese Coney' w/onions, extra long	1 serving	640	25	47	632	0	39.2	65.0	0	55%
'Cheese Coney' regular	1 serving	358	14	23	341	0	23.3	40.0	0	59%
regular	1 serving	258	8	21	241	0	15.3	23.0	0	54%
'Cheese Coney' regular, w/onions	1 serving	361	14	24	341	0	23.3	40.0	0	58%
SANDWICH										
bacon, lettuce, tomato	1 sandwich	327	8	27	600	0	19.3	9.0	0	56%
cheese, grilled	1 sandwich	288	12	25	841	0	17.0	36.0	0	51%
chicken	1 sandwich	319	21	41	890	0	9.0	47.0	0	25%
chicken, breaded	1 sandwich	455	23	36	755	0	24.7	42.0	0	48%
chicken, grilled, no dressing	1 sandwich	215	21	23	716	0	4.3	63.0	0	18%
fish	1 sandwich	277	17	38	655	0	7.0	6.0	0	22%
steak	1 sandwich	631	19	46	1047	0	41.6	50.0	0	59%
SIDE DISH										
french fries, large	1 serving	315	5	50	67	0	11.2	11.0	0	32%
french fries, regular	1 serving	233	3	37	50	0	8.0	8.0	0	31%
french fries, w/cheese, large	1 serving	420	11	51	468	0	20.2	38.0	0	43%
onion rings, large	1 serving	577	8	54	532	0	37.8	0.0	0	58%
onion rings, regular	1 serving	404	5	38	372	0	26.5	0.0	0	58%
potato pieces, 'Tater Tots'	1 serving	150	2	19	330	0	7.0	10.0	0	43%
potato pieces, 'Tater Tots' w/cheese	1 serving	220	6	19	569	0	13.0	28.0	0	54%

SPAGHETTI WAREHOUSE

Food Name	Serv. Size	Total Cal.	Prot. gms	Carbs gms	Sod. mgs	Fiber gms	Fat gms	Chol. mgs	Sat.Fat gms	%Fat Cal.
MARINADE, dinner serving	1 serving	403	13	75	303	5	5.0	0.0	0	11%
MINESTRONE SOUP	1 serving	56	3	8	155	2	1.0	3.0	0	17%
TOMATO SAUCE, dinner serving	1 serving	410	13	76	454	6	5.0	0.0	0	11%

STEAK 'N SHAKE
CHEESEBURGER

Food Name	Serv. Size	Total Cal.	Prot. gms	Carbs gms	Sod. mgs	Fiber gms	Fat gms	Chol. mgs	Sat.Fat gms	%Fat Cal.
'Steakburger'	1 serving	353	23	33	658	0	13.0	0.0	0	34%
'Steakburger' super	1 serving	451	35	33	680	0	18.0	0.0	0	37%
'Steakburger' triple patty	1 serving	626	52	34	934	0	30.0	0.0	0	44%
CHILI										
'Chili Mac' w/4 saltines	1 serving	310	15	34	1301	0	12.0	0.0	0	36%
'Chili 3 Ways' w/4 saltines	1 serving	411	19	45	1734	0	16.0	0.0	0	36%
w/oyster crackers	1 serving	337	16	37	1157	0	14.0	0.0	0	37%
DESSERT										
apple Danish	1 piece	391	6	35	352	0	24.0	0.0	0	57%
apple pie à la mode	1 serving	549	4	76	525	0	25.0	0.0	0	41%
brownie	1 brownie	258	3	39	165	0	12.0	0.0	0	39%
cheesecake	1 serving	368	7	61	294	0	11.0	0.0	0	27%
cheesecake, w/strawberries	1 serving	386	7	65	294	0	11.0	0.0	0	26%
cherry pie à la mode'	1 serving	476	6	63	314	0	22.0	0.0	0	42%
'Coca-Cola Float'	1 serving	514	16	76	230	0	17.0	0.0	0	29%
fudge brownie sundae	1 serving	645	7	81	262	0	35.0	0.0	0	47%
hot fudge nut sundae	1 serving	530	5	51	121	0	34.0	0.0	0	58%

Food Name	Serv. Size	Total Cal.	Prot. gms	Carbs gms	Sod. mgs	Fiber gms	Fat gms	Chol. mgs	Sat.Fat gms	%Fat Cal.
'Lemon Float'	1 serving	555	18	82	248	0	19.0	0.0	0	30%
'Lemon Freeze'	1 serving	548	15	69	213	0	25.0	0.0	0	40%
'Orange Float'	1 serving	502	16	74	224	0	17.0	0.0	0	30%
'Orange Freeze'	1 serving	516	14	63	198	0	24.0	0.0	0	41%
'Root Beer Float'	1 serving	529	17	78	237	0	17.0	0.0	0	29%
strawberry sundae	1 serving	330	2	29	81	0	22.0	0.0	0	61%
HAMBURGER										
'Steakburger'	1 serving	277	18	33	425	0	7.0	0.0	0	24%
'Steakburger' super	1 serving	375	30	33	447	0	12.0	0.0	0	30%
'Steakburger' triple patty	1 serving	474	43	33	468	0	17.0	0.0	0	33%
SALAD										
chef	1 salad	313	41	6	1582	0	18.0	0.0	0	46%
lettuce and tomato, w/1 oz Thousand Island dressing	1 salad	168	1	7	223	0	15.0	0.0	0	81%
SANDWICH										
cheese, toasted	1 sandwich	250	9	24	606	0	13.0	0.0	0	47%
egg	1 sandwich	275	12	33	490	0	10.0	0.0	0	33%
ham, baked	1 sandwich	451	29	37	1858	0	22.0	0.0	0	43%
ham and egg	1 sandwich	434	36	33	1850	0	17.0	0.0	0	36%
SIDE DISH										
baked beans	1 serving	173	9	27	656	0	4.0	0.0	0	20%
french fries	1 serving	211	3	28	297	0	10.0	0.0	0	42%
STEAK PLATTER, low calorie	1 serving	293	37	3	242	0	14.0	0.0	0	44%
SUBWAY										
BEVERAGE										
'Berry 'Lishus Fruizle Smoothie'	12 oz	154	1	40	9	3	0.3	0.0	0	2%
'Berry Blitz Fruizle Smoothie'	12 oz	129	1	37	7	7	0.0	0.0	0	0%
'Berry Breeze Fruizle Smoothie'	12 oz	120	0	32	7	2	0.1	0.0	0	1%
'Island Berry Fruizle Smoothie'	12 oz	120	0	32	7	2	0.1	0.0	0	1%
'Island Fever Fruizle Smoothie'	12 oz	137	0	36	7	1	0.2	0.0	0	1%
'Peach Paradise Fruizle Smoothie'	12 oz	119	0	32	7	1	0.1	0.0	0	1%
'Peach Pizazz Fruizle Smoothie'	12 oz	126	0	33	10	1	0.0	0.0	0	0%
'Pineapple Delite Fruizle Smoothie'	12 oz	142	1	38	6	1	0.3	0.0	0	2%
'Pineapple Passion Fruizle Smoothie'	12 oz	140	1	38	6	1	0.2	0.0	0	1%
'Sunrise Energizer Fruizle Smoothie'	12 oz	160	1	42	8	2	0.3	0.0	0	2%
'Tropical Trio Fruizle Smoothie'	12 oz	138	0	36	7	1	0.2	0.0	0	1%
'Wild Berries Fruizle Smoothie'	12 oz	130	1	36	8	5	0.1	0.0	0	1%
BREAD										
Italian, 12-inch	1 large	380	14	76	840	0	2.0	0.0	2	5%
Italian, 6-inch	1 small	190	7	38	420	0	1.0	0.0	1	5%
wheat, 12-inch	1 serving	420	16	78	860	6	5.0	0.0	2	11%
wheat, 6-inch	1 serving	210	8	39	430	3	3.0	0.0	1	13%
wrap, 10.5-inch	1 wrap	200	0	45	720	1	2.0	0.0	1	9%
CONDIMENTS										
bacon, 'Optional Fixin's'	2 slices	42	3	0	160	0	3.0	9.0	1	69%
cheese	2 triangles	41	2	0	204	0	3.0	10.0	2	77%
lettuce, deli style, 'Standard Fixin's'	1 serving	2	0	0	1	0	0.0	0.0	0	0%
lettuce, 'Standard Fixin's'	1 serving	4	0	1	3	0	0.0	0.0	0	0%
mayonnaise, light, 'Optional Fixin's'	1 tsp	18	0	0	33	0	2.0	2.0	0	100%
mayonnaise, regular, 'Optional Fixin's'	1 tsp	37	0	0	27	0	4.0	3.0	1	100%

Food Name	Serv. Size	Total Cal.	Prot. gms	Carbs gms	Sod. mgs	Fiber gms	Fat gms	Chol. mgs	Sat.Fat gms	%Fat Cal.
vinegar, 'Optional Fixin's'	1 tsp	1	0	0	0	0	0.0	0.0	0	0%
mustard, 'Optional Fixin's'	2 tsp	7	0	1	115	0	0.0	0.0	0	0%
oil, 'Optional Fixin's'	1 tsp	45	0	0	0	0	5.0	0.0	1	100%
olives, deli style, 'Standard Fixin's'	2 rings	2	0	0	6	0	0.0	0.0	0	0%
olives, 'Standard Fixin's'	2 rings	2	0	0	6	0	0.0	0.0	0	0%
onion, deli style, 'Standard Fixin's'	1 serving	2	0	1	0	0	0.0	0.0	0	0%
onion 'Standard Fixin's'	1 serving	5	0	1	0	0	0.0	0.0	0	0%
peppers, deli style 'Standard Fixin's'	2 strips	1	0	0	0	na	0.0	0.0	0	0%
peppers, 'Standard Fixin's'	2 strips	1	0	0	0	0	0.0	0.0	0	0%
pickle, deli style, 'Standard Fixin's'	2 chips	1	0	0	92	0	0.0	0.0	0	0%
pickle, 'Standard Fixin's'	3 chips	2	0	0	139	0	0.0	0.0	0	0%
tomato, deli style, 'Standard Fixin's'	2 slices	8	0	2	4	0	0.0	0.0	0	0%
tomato, 'Standard Fixin's'	2 slices	6	0	1	2	0	0.0	0.0	0	0%
COOKIE										
Brazil nut	1 cookie	215	2	29	153	1	10.0	14.0	3	42%
chocolate chip, 'M&M's	1 cookie	212	2	29	144	1	10.0	13.0	3	42%
chocolate chip	1 cookie	214	3	29	144	1	10.0	12.0	3	41%
chocolate chunk	1 cookie	215	2	29	144	1	10.0	13.0	3	42%
macadamia nut	1 cookie	222	2	28	144	1	11.0	12.0	2	45%
oatmeal raisin	1 cookie	199	3	29	159	1	8.0	14.0	2	36%
oatmeal raisin, low-fat	1 cookie	168	3	33	171	2	3.0	15.0	1	16%
peanut butter	1 cookie	223	3	27	214	1	12.0	0.0	2	47%
sugar	1 cookie	225	2	28	180	0	12.0	18.0	3	47%
ROLL, deli style	1 serving	170	6	31	350	1	2.0	0.0	1	11%
SALAD										
chicken breast, roasted, w/o dressing, cheese, condiments	1 salad	162	20	13	693	1	4.0	48.0	1	21%
'Classic Italian BMT, w/o dressing, cheese, condiments	1 salad	269	14	11	1305	1	19.0	52.0	7	63%
'Cold Cut Trio' w/o dressing, cheese, condiments	1 salad	193	12	12	1162	1	12.0	47.0	4	53%
ham, w/o dressing, cheese, condiments	1 salad	112	12	11	1068	1	3.0	25.0	1	23%
meatball, w/o dressing, cheese, ondiments	1 salad	232	13	17	751	3	13.0	35.0	5	49%
roast beef, w/o dressing, cheese, condiments	1 salad	115	12	11	654	1	3.0	20.0	1	23%
seafood and crab, w/light mayo, w/o dressing	1 salad	157	7	17	761	2	7.0	14.0	1	40%
steak and cheese, w/o dressing	1 salad	182	17	13	887	2	8.0	37.0	4	38%
'Subway Club' w/o dressing, cheese, condiments	1 salad	123	14	12	965	1	3.0	26.0	1	21%
'Subway Melt' w/o dressing	1 salad	190	16	12	1346	1	9.0	41.0	4	42%
tuna, made w/light mayo, w/o dressing, cheese, condiments	1 salad	198	11	11	669	1	12.0	32.0	2	55%
turkey and ham, w/o dressing, cheese, condiments	1 salad	107	11	11	982	1	2.0	23.0	1	17%
turkey breast, w/o dressing, cheese, condiments	1 salad	101	11	12	896	1	2.0	20.0	0	16%

Food Name	Serv. Size	Total Cal.	Prot. gms	Carbs gms	Sod. mgs	Fiber gms	Fat gms	Chol. mgs	Sat.Fat gms	%Fat Cal.
'Veggie Delite,' w/o dressing, cheese, condiments .... 1 salad		51	2	10	308	1	1.0	0.0	0	16%
SANDWICH										
Bacon and egg										
deli style sub .... 1 sandwich		323	14	33	569	1	14.0	185.0	4	40%
6-inch sub .... 1 sandwich		363	16	41	649	3	15.0	185.0	4	37%
wrap .... 1 sandwich		353	8	47	939	1	14.0	185.0	4	36%
Bologna, deli style sub, w/o cheese, condiments .... 1 sandwich		283	11	37	785	1	10.0	19.0	3	32%
Cheese and egg										
deli style sub .... 1 sandwich		323	14	33	613	1	14.0	187.0	5	40%
6-inch sub .... 1 sandwich		363	16	41	693	3	15.0	187.0	5	37%
wrap .... 1 sandwich		353	8	47	983	1	14.0	187.0	5	36%
Chicken breast										
roasted, 6-inch hot sub, w/o cheese, condiments .... 1 sandwich		342	26	46	966	3	6.0	48.0	2	16%
roasted, super, 6-inch hot sub, w/o cheese, condiments .... 1 sandwich		453	44	49	1351	4	9.0	96.0	3	18%
Chicken Parmesan wrap .... 1 sandwich		333	17	56	1393	2	5.0	45.0	2	13%
'Classic Italian BMT'										
6-inch sub, w/o cheese, condiments .... 1 sandwich		450	21	45	1579	3	21.0	52.0	8	42%
super, 6-inch sub, w/o cheese, condiments .... 1 sandwich		668	33	47	2576	3	39.0	104.0	354	52%
'Cold Cut Trio'										
6-inch sub, w/o cheese, condiments .... 1 sandwich		374	19	45	1435	3	14.0	47.0	5	33%
super, 6-inch sub, w/o cheese, condiments .... 1 sandwich		517	29	47	2289	3	24.0	93.0	220	42%
Ham and egg										
deli style sub .... 1 sandwich		312	16	33	789	1	12.0	189.0	3	36%
6-inch sub .... 1 sandwich		352	18	41	869	3	13.0	189.0	3	33%
wrap .... 1 sandwich		342	10	47	1159	1	12.0	189.0	3	32%
Ham										
deli style sub, w/o cheese, condiments .... 1 sandwich		224	12	37	827	1	3.0	12.0	0	12%
6-inch sub, w/o cheese, condiments .... 1 sandwich		293	18	45	1342	3	5.0	25.0	2	15%
super, 6-inch sub, w/o cheese, condiments .... 1 sandwich		354	27	47	2101	3	7.0	50.0	60	18%
Meatball										
6-inch hot sub, w/o cheese, condiments .... 1 sandwich		413	19	50	1025	5	15.0	35.0	6	33%
super, 6-inch hot sub, w/o cheese, condiments .... 1 sandwich		594	30	58	1468	7	27.0	70.0	11	41%
Roast beef										
deli style sub, w/o cheese, condiments .... 1 sandwich		236	14	37	678	1	4.0	13.0	0	15%

Food Name	Serv. Size	Total Cal.	Prot. gms	Carbs gms	Sod. mgs	Fiber gms	Fat gms	Chol. mgs	Sat.Fat gms	%Fat Cal.
6-inch sub, w/o cheese, condiments	1 sandwich	296	19	45	928	3	5.0	20.0	2	15%
super, 6-inch sub, w/o cheese, condiments	1 sandwich	360	29	47	1273	3	7.0	40.0	61	17%
Seafood and crab										
super, w/light mayo, 6-inch sub	1 sandwich	444	18	58	1486	5	15.0	27.0	137	31%
w/light mayo, 6-inch sub	1 sandwich	338	14	51	1034	4	9.0	14.0	2	24%
Steak and cheese										
6-inch hot sub	1 sandwich	363	24	47	1160	4	10.0	37.0	4	24%
super, 6-inch sub	1 sandwich	495	39	50	1739	5	17.0	75.0	8	30%
wrap	1 sandwich	353	16	53	1450	2	9.0	37.0	4	23%
'Subway Club'										
6-inch sub, w/o cheese, condiments	1 sandwich	304	21	46	1239	3	5.0	26.0	2	14%
super, 6-inch sub, w/o cheese, condiments	1 sandwich	377	32	48	1895	3	7.0	52.0	59	16%
'Subway Melt'										
6-inch hot sub	1 sandwich	370	23	46	1619	3	11.0	41.0	5	26%
super, 6-inch hot sub	1 sandwich	509	36	48	2657	3	19.0	83.0	9	34%
Tuna										
w/light mayo, deli style sub, w/o cheese, condiments	1 sandwich	267	12	37	627	1	8.0	16.0	1	27%
w/light mayo, 6-inch sub, w/o cheese, condiments	1 sandwich	378	18	45	942	3	14.0	32.0	3	33%
w/light mayo, super, 6-inch sub, w/o cheese, condiments	1 sandwich	525	27	46	1303	3	26.0	64.0	5	44%
Turkey and ham										
6-inch sub, w/o cheese, condiments	1 sandwich	288	18	45	1256	3	4.0	23.0	2	13%
super, 6-inch sub, w/o cheese, condiments	1 sandwich	343	27	47	1929	3	6.0	45.0	50	15%
Turkey bacon wrap, deluxe	1 sandwich	355	14	52	1823	1	10.0	39.0	4	25%
Turkey breast										
deli style sub, w/o cheese, condiments	1 sandwich	227	13	37	678	1	4.0	13.0	0	15%
6-inch sub, w/o cheese, condiments	1 sandwich	282	17	45	1170	3	4.0	20.0	1	13%
super, 6-inch sub, w/o cheese, condiments	1 sandwich	333	26	47	1758	3	4.0	40.0	40	11%
'Veggie Delite' 6-inch sub, w/o cheese, condiments	1 sandwich	232	9	43	582	3	3.0	0.0	1	11%
Western egg										
deli style sub	1 sandwich	311	14	36	603	2	12.0	182.0	3	35%
6-inch sub	1 sandwich	351	16	44	683	4	12.0	182.0	3	31%
wrap	1 sandwich	341	8	50	973	2	12.0	182.0	3	32%

SWENSEN'S
ICE CREAM

Food Name	Serv. Size	Total Cal.	Prot. gms	Carbs gms	Sod. mgs	Fiber gms	Fat gms	Chol. mgs	Sat.Fat gms	%Fat Cal.
'Almond Praline Delight' low-fat	1/2 cup	130	3	25	85	0	2.0	5.0	1	14%
caramel apple crisp, low-fat	1/2 cup	130	3	26	75	0	1.0	5.0	1	7%

Food Name	Serv. Size	Total Cal.	Prot. gms	Carbs gms	Sod. mgs	Fiber gms	Fat gms	Chol. mgs	Sat.Fat gms	%Fat Cal.
caramel turtle fudge, light	1 serving	120	3	18	50	0	4.0	10.0	0	30%
caramel turtle fudge, low-fat	1/2 cup	140	3	26	70	0	2.5	5.0	1	16%
chocolate chocolate chip cheesecake, low-fat	1/2 cup	130	3	26	80	0	2.5	5.0	1	16%
chocolate fudge brownie, low-fat	1/2 cup	120	3	24	70	0	2.5	5.0	1	17%
cookies and cream, light	1 serving	130	3	20	60	0	4.0	10.0	0	28%
ice cream, cookies and cream, low-fat	1/2 cup	130	3	25	80	0	2.5	5.0	1	17%
vanilla, light	1 serving	110	3	15	50	0	4.0	10.0	0	33%
YOGURT, FROZEN										
Black Forest cake	1 serving	95	3	21	130	0	1.0	5.0	0	9%
Black Forest cake, low-fat	1/2 cup	110	4	22	55	1	1.5	0.0	1	11%
blueberry and cream, gourmet, sugar-free	1 serving	110	3	17	90	0	4.0	10.0	0	31%
butter pecan, low-fat	1/2 cup	120	4	20	55	0	3.0	5.0	1	22%
cherry, nonfat	1/2 cup	90	3	20	45	0	0.0	0.0	0	0%
chocolate raspberry truffle, gourmet, sugar-free	1 serving	130	3	18	80	0	5.0	8.0	0	35%
coconut pineapple	1 serving	120	4	26	65	0	1.0	5.0	0	7%
hazelnut amaretto, low-fat	1/2 cup	120	4	20	50	0	3.0	0.0	0	22%
mocha chip, low-fat	1/2 cup	110	4	22	50	0	1.5	0.0	1	11%
strawberry banana and cream, nonfat	1/2 cup	90	3	20	45	0	0.0	0.0	0	0%
triple chocolate, low-fat	1/2 cup	120	4	24	50	1	1.5	0.0	1	11%
triple chocolate, nonfat	1 serving	100	4	21	65	0	0.0	0.0	0	0%
vanilla, nonfat	1/2 cup	90	3	20	60	0	0.0	0.0	0	0%
vanilla Swiss almond, gourmet, sugar-free	1 serving	140	4	15	100	0	7.0	10.0	0	45%

SWISS CHALET

Food Name	Serv. Size	Total Cal.	Prot. gms	Carbs gms	Sod. mgs	Fiber gms	Fat gms	Chol. mgs	Sat.Fat gms	%Fat Cal.
CHICKEN	1/2 chicken	634	72	1	0	0	38.0	0.0	0	54%
DESSERT										
apple pie	1 serving	394	3	45	0	0	23.0	0.0	0	52%
Black Forest cake	1 piece	278	3	36	0	0	14.0	0.0	0	45%
chocolate éclair	1 serving	205	2	27	0	0	10.0	0.0	0	44%
coconut pie	1 serving	292	2	40	0	0	14.0	0.0	0	43%
fudge nut cake	1 piece	346	4	48	0	0	16.0	0.0	0	41%
vanilla ice cream	1 serving	195	3	16	0	0	14.0	0.0	0	62%
GRAVY, sandwich	1 serving	35	1	5	0	0	1.0	0.0	0	27%
ROLL	1 roll	116	3	24	0	0	1.0	0.0	0	8%
SALAD, chicken	1 salad	500	42	23	0	0	42.0	0.0	0	59%
SANDWICH										
chicken	1 sandwich	360	33	42	0	0	5.0	0.0	0	13%
chicken, hot	1 sandwich	310	30	30	0	0	6.0	0.0	0	18%
SIDE DISH										
baked potato	1 serving	227	8	52	0	0	0.0	0.0	0	0%
coleslaw, 'Chalet'	1 serving	56	2	10	0	0	1.0	0.0	0	16%
french fries	1 serving	478	10	57	0	0	24.0	0.0	0	45%
SOUP, chicken, 'Chalet'	1 serving	97	9	11	0	0	2.0	0.0	0	18%

TCBY
YOGURT, FROZEN

Food Name	Serv. Size	Total Cal.	Prot. gms	Carbs gms	Sod. mgs	Fiber gms	Fat gms	Chol. mgs	Sat.Fat gms	%Fat Cal.
nonfat, giant	31.6 oz	869	32	182	356	0	0.0	0.0	0	0%

Food Name	Serv. Size	Total Cal.	Prot. gms	Carbs gms	Sod. mgs	Fiber gms	Fat gms	Chol. mgs	Sat.Fat gms	%Fat Cal.
nonfat, kiddie	3.2 oz	88	3	18	36	0	0.0	0.0	0	0%
nonfat, large	10.5 oz	289	10	60	118	0	0.0	0.0	0	0%
nonfat, medium	8.2 oz	226	8	47	92	0	0.0	0.0	0	0%
nonfat, small	5.9 oz	162	6	34	66	0	0.0	0.0	0	0%
nonfat, super	15.2 oz	418	15	87	171	0	0.0	0.0	0	0%
regular, giant	31.6 oz	1027	32	182	474	0	24.0	79.0	16	20%
regular, kiddie	3.2 oz	104	3	18	48	0	2.0	8.0	2	18%
regular, large	10.5 oz	342	10	60	156	0	8.0	26.0	5	20%
regular, medium	8.2 oz	267	8	47	126	0	6.0	20.0	4	20%
regular, small	5.9 oz	192	6	34	90	0	4.0	15.0	3	18%
regular, super	15.2 oz	494	15	87	228	0	11.0	38.0	8	20%
strawberry	8 oz	220	9	43	150	0	2.0	0.0	0	8%
sugarless, nonfat, giant	31.6 oz	632	32	142	316	0	0.0	0.0	0	0%
sugarless, nonfat, kiddie	3.2 oz	64	3	14	32	0	0.0	0.0	0	0%
sugarless, nonfat, large	10.5 oz	210	10	47	105	0	0.0	0.0	0	0%
sugarless, nonfat, medium	8.2 oz	164	8	37	82	0	0.0	0.0	0	0%
sugarless, nonfat, small	5.9 oz	118	6	27	59	0	0.0	0.0	0	0%
sugarless, nonfat, super	15.2 oz	304	15	68	152	0	0.0	0.0	0	0%
TACO BELL										
BURRITO										
bacon and egg, double, 6.25 oz	1 serving	480	18	39	1240	2	27.0	400.0	9	52%
bean, 7 oz	1 serving	370	13	54	1080	12	12.0	10.0	4	29%
'Big Beef' 7 oz	1 serving	400	19	43	1320	6	17.0	50.0	6	38%
'Big Beef Supreme' 10.5 oz	1 serving	510	23	52	1500	11	23.0	60.0	9	41%
'Big Chicken Supreme' 9 oz	1 serving	460	27	50	1200	3	17.0	70.0	6	33%
chicken, grilled, 7 oz	1 serving	390	19	49	1240	3	13.0	40.0	4	30%
chili cheese, 5 oz	1 serving	330	13	40	900	4	13.0	25.0	5	36%
'Country Breakfast' 4 oz	1 serving	270	8	26	690	2	14.0	195.0	5	48%
'Fiesta Breakfast' 3.5 oz	1 serving	280	9	25	580	2	16.0	25.0	6	51%
'Grande Breakfast' 6.25 oz	1 serving	420	13	43	1050	3	22.0	205.0	7	47%
7-layer, 10 oz	1 serving	520	16	65	1270	13	22.0	25.0	7	38%
'Supreme' 9 oz	1 serving	430	17	50	1210	9	18.0	40.0	7	38%
CHALUPA										
'Baja Beef' 5.5 oz	1 serving	420	14	30	760	3	27.0	35.0	7	58%
'Baja Chicken' 5.5 oz	1 serving	400	17	28	660	2	24.0	40.0	5	55%
'Baja Steak' 5.5 oz	1 serving	400	17	27	680	2	24.0	30.0	6	55%
beef, supreme, 5.5 oz	1 serving	380	14	29	580	3	23.0	40.0	8	55%
chicken, supreme, 5.5 oz	1 serving	360	17	28	490	2	20.0	45.0	7	50%
'Santa Fe Beef' 5.5 oz	1 serving	440	14	31	660	4	29.0	35.0	7	59%
'Santa Fe Chicken' 5.5 oz	1 serving	420	17	30	560	2	26.0	40.0	6	55%
'Santa Fe Steak' 5.5 oz	1 serving	430	18	29	580	2	27.0	35.0	6	56%
steak, supreme, 5.5 oz	1 serving	360	17	27	500	2	20.0	35.0	7	51%
CINNAMON TWIST, 1 oz	1 serving	180	1	25	290	1	8.0	0.0	2	41%
DESSERT, choco taco ice cream, 4 oz	1 serving	310	3	37	100	1	17.0	20.0	10	49%
GORDITA										
'Baja Beef' 5.5 oz	1 serving	360	13	29	810	4	21.0	35.0	5	53%
'Baja Chicken' 5.5 oz	1 serving	340	16	28	710	3	18.0	40.0	4	48%
'Baja Steak' 5.5 oz	1 serving	340	17	27	730	3	18.0	30.0	4	48%
beef, supreme, 5.5 oz	1 serving	300	17	27	550	3	14.0	35.0	5	42%
chicken, supreme, 5.5 oz	1 serving	300	16	28	530	3	13.0	45.0	5	40%

Food Name	Serv. Size	Total Cal.	Prot. gms	Carbs gms	Sod. mgs	Fiber gms	Fat gms	Chol. mgs	Sat.Fat gms	%Fat Cal.
'Santa Fe Beef' 5.5 oz .... 1 serving		380	14	31	700	5	23.0	35.0	5	53%
'Santa Fe Chicken' 5.5 oz .... 1 serving		370	17	30	610	3	20.0	40.0	4	49%
'Santa Fe Steak' 5.5 oz .... 1 serving		370	17	29	620	3	20.0	35.0	5	49%
steak, supreme, 5.5 oz .... 1 serving		300	17	27	550	3	14.0	35.0	5	42%
MEXIMELT, big beef, 4.75 oz .... 1 serving		290	15	22	830	4	15.0	45.0	7	48%
NACHOS										
'Bellegrande' 11 oz .... 1 serving		760	20	83	1300	17	39.0	35.0	11	46%
'Big Beef Supreme' 7 oz .... 1 serving		440	14	44	800	9	24.0	35.0	7	48%
chicken, 'Bellegrande' 11 oz .... 1 serving		740	23	82	1200	15	36.0	40.0	9	44%
regular, 3.5 oz .... 1 serving		320	5	34	560	3	18.0	5.0	4	51%
steak, 'Bellegrande' 11 oz .... 1 serving		740	24	81	1220	15	37.0	35.0	9	44%
PIZZA										
Mexican, 7.75 oz .... 1 serving		540	20	42	1030	7	35.0	45.0	10	56%
Mexican beef, 7.75 oz .... 1 serving		530	24	39	950	6	33.0	45.0	9	54%
Mexican chicken, 7.75 oz .... 1 serving		520	23	41	940	6	32.0	50.0	8	53%
QUESADILLA										
cheese, 4.25 oz ...../............ 1 serving		350	16	31	860	3	18.0	50.0	9	46%
cheese, breakfast, 5.5 oz .... 1 serving		380	15	33	1010	1	21.0	280.0	9	50%
chicken, 6 oz .... 1 serving		400	25	33	1050	3	19.0	75.0	9	42%
w/bacon, breakfast, 6 oz .... 1 serving		450	19	33	1200	2	27.0	290.0	11	54%
w/sausage, breakfast, 6 oz .... 1 serving		430	17	33	1090	1	25.0	285.0	10	53%
SALAD										
taco, w/salsa, 19 oz .... 1 salad		850	30	69	2250	16	52.0	70.0	14	54%
taco, w/salsa, w/o shell, 16.5 oz .... 1 salad		430	25	36	1990	15	22.0	70.0	10	45%
SIDE DISH										
hash brown nuggets, 3.5 oz .... 1 serving		280	2	29	570	1	18.0	0.0	5	57%
Mexican rice, 4.75 oz .... 1 serving		190	5	23	750	1	9.0	15.0	4	42%
pintos and cheese, 4.5 oz .... 1 serving		180	9	18	640	10	8.0	15.0	4	40%
TACO										
'Double Decker' 5.75 oz .... 1 serving		330	14	37	740	9	15.0	30.0	5	40%
'Double Decker Supreme' 7 oz .... 1 serving		380	15	39	760	9	18.0	40.0	7	43%
'Supreme' 4 oz.................... 1 serving		210	9	14	350	3	14.0	40.0	6	58%
grilled chicken, soft, 4.5 oz .... 1 serving		200	14	20	530	2	7.0	35.0	3	32%
grilled steak, soft, 4.5 oz .... 1 serving		200	14	19	570	2	7.0	25.0	3	32%
grilled steak, soft, 'Supreme' 5.75 oz ... 1 serving		240	15	21	580	2	11.0	35.0	5	41%
regular, 2.75 oz .... 1 serving		170	9	12	340	3	10.0	30.0	4	52%
soft, 'Supreme' 5 oz .... 1 serving		260	11	22	590	3	13.0	40.0	6	47%
soft, 3.5 oz....................... 1 serving		210	11	20	570	3	10.0	30.0	4	42%
TOSTADA, 6.25 oz .... 1 serving		250	10	27	640	11	12.0	15.0	5	42%

TACO JOHN'S
BURRITO

Food Name	Serv. Size	Total Cal.	Prot. gms	Carbs gms	Sod. mgs	Fiber gms	Fat gms	Chol. mgs	Sat.Fat gms	%Fat Cal.
bean .... 5 oz		249	10	36	636	0	6.0	0.0	0	23%
beef .... 5 oz		355	16	25	666	0	18.0	0.0	0	50%
chicken, super, w/o sour cream,										
cheese .... 1 serving		366	30	40	844	0	14.0	0.0	0	31%
chicken, w/o sour cream, cheese ...... 1 serving		227	27	19	639	0	10.0	0.0	0	33%
combination .... 5 oz		302	11	30	651	0	12.0	0.0	0	40%
super .... 8.3 oz		434	17	66	1022	0	11.0	0.0	0	23%

Food Name	Serv. Size	Total Cal.	Prot. gms	Carbs gms	Sod. mgs	Fiber gms	Fat gms	Chol. mgs	Sat.Fat gms	%Fat Cal.
super, w/o sour cream, cheese .... 1 serving		389	18	51	856	0	16.0	0.0	0	34%
Texas chili .... 12.3 oz		518	23	48	746	0	24.0	0.0	0	43%
w/green chili .... 12.3 oz		405	18	38	995	0	24.0	0.0	0	49%
w/green chili, w/o sour cream, cheese .... 1 serving		367	20	40	998	0	18.0	0.0	0	40%
CHILI, Texas .... 9.5 oz		430	23	35	1580	0	22.0	0.0	0	46%
CHIMICHANGA .... 12 oz		487	16	54	1226	0	19.0	0.0	0	38%
ENCHILADA .... 7 oz		379	19	33	431	0	18.0	0.0	0	44%
NACHOS										
regular .... 4 oz		407	11	42	307	0	19.0	0.0	0	45%
super .... 11.25 oz		657	23	57	857	0	34.0	0.0	0	49%
PASTRY										
'Apple Grande' Danish .... 3 oz		257	5	44	231	0	8.0	0.0	0	27%
churro .... 1.2 oz		122	2	12	153	0	7.0	0.0	0	53%
SALAD										
chicken taco, super, w/o dressing, sour cream .... 1 salad		377	26	56	882	0	15.0	0.0	0	29%
taco, w/o shell, dressing, sour cream, cheese .... 1 salad		228	13	30	440	0	13.0	0.0	0	40%
taco, super .... 12.3 oz		450	16	48	880	0	18.0	0.0	0	39%
SANDWICH, chicken fillet, 'Sierra' .... 8.5 oz		500	31	46	1493	23	21.0	41.0	0	38%
SIDE DISH										
'Potato Ole' large .... 6 oz		414	6	96	1595	0	6.0	0.0	0	12%
refried beans .... 9.5 oz		331	19	79	1195	0	6.0	0.0	0	12%
Mexican rice .... 1 serving		340	7	59	1280	0	8.0	0.0	0	21%
TACO										
'Taco Bravo' w/o sour cream .... 1 serving		319	16	42	658	0	14.0	0.0	0	35%
'Taco Bravo' super .... 8 oz		485	18	51	1006	0	20.0	0.0	0	39%
chicken, soft shell .... 1 serving		180	18	20	490	0	8.0	0.0	0	32%
regular .... 4.3 oz		228	11	15	347	0	13.0	0.0	0	53%
soft .... 5 oz		276	13	23	505	0	13.0	0.0	0	45%
TACOBURGER .... 6 oz		332	14	31	660	0	14.0	0.0	0	41%
TOSTADA .... 4.3 oz		228	11	15	347	0	13.0	0.0	0	53%
TACO TIME										
BEEF, shredded .... 2.5 oz		70	1	1	31	0	0.0	0.0	0	0%
BURRITO										
bean, crisp .... 5.25 oz		427	15	53	453	9	18.0	12.0	5	37%
bean, soft, double .... 9.5 oz		506	23	77	860	19	12.0	22.0	6	21%
bean, soft, single, 'Value' .... 6.75 oz		380	16	58	715	13	10.0	15.0	4	23%
chicken, crisp .... 4.75 oz		422	17	32	795	2	25.0	54.0	8	53%
combination, soft, double .... 9.5 oz		617	39	66	1343	18	23.0	63.0	10	33%
meat, 'Casita' .... 12 oz		647	40	54	1233	16	31.0	89.0	15	43%
meat, crisp .... 5.25 oz		552	34	39	1000	7	30.0	58.0	10	48%
meat, soft, double .... 9.5 oz		726	57	55	1809	17	33.0	99.0	14	40%
meat, soft, single, 'Value' .... 6.75 oz		491	31	48	1197	12	21.0	56.0	8	37%
veggie .... 11 oz		491	21	70	643	10	16.0	24.0	6	28%
CHEESE, Cheddar .... 0.75 oz		86	5	0	132	0	7.0	22.0	4	76%
CHEESEBURGER, taco, meat .... 7.5 oz		633	31	48	1291	7	36.0	66.0	10	51%
CHICKEN .... 2.5 oz		109	11	2	402	0	6.0	33.0	2	51%

Food Name	Serv. Size	Total Cal.	Prot. gms	Carbs gms	Sod. mgs	Fiber gms	Fat gms	Chol. mgs	Sat.Fat gms	%Fat Cal.
CHIPS	2 oz	266	4	35	461	3	12.0	0.0	3	41%
CRUSTOS	3.5 oz	373	9	47	86	na	15.0	0.0	na	38%
CONDIMENTS										
enchilada sauce	1 oz	12	0	3	133	1	0.0	0.0	0	0%
guacamole	1 oz	29	0	2	94	1	2.0	0.0	0	69%
hot sauce	1 oz	10	0	2	120	0	0.0	0.0	0	0%
salad dressing, sour cream	1.5 oz	137	1	2	207	0	14.0	8.0	5	91%
salad dressing, Thousand Island	1 oz	160	0	4	220	0	16.0	10.0	2	90%
salsa, ranchero	2 oz	21	1	3	192	1	1.0	0.0	0	36%
sour cream	1 oz	55	1	1	11	0	5.0	19.0	3	85%
EMPANADA, cherry	4 oz	250	5	37	46	na	9.0	0.0	na	33%
LETTUCE	0.5 oz	2	0	0	1	0	0.0	0.0	0	0%
NACHOS										
deluxe	15.25 oz	1048	46	91	2252	17	57.0	109.0	23	48%
regular	10.5 oz	680	26	61	1250	11	38.0	78.0	19	50%
QUESADILLA, cheese	3.25 oz	205	11	17	255	1	11.0	30.0	6	47%
SALAD										
chicken taco, w/o dressing	9 oz	370	19	27	861	3	21.0	48.0	7	51%
taco, regular, w/o dressing	7.5 oz	479	30	30	895	7	28.0	63.0	11	51%
'Tostada Delight' w/meat	9.75 oz	628	36	48	1004	13	33.0	82.0	14	47%
SIDE DISH										
french fries, 'Mexi'	8 oz	532	6	54	1598	na	34.0	0.0	na	56%
french fries, 'Mexi' regular	4 oz	266	3	27	799	na	17.0	0.0	na	56%
Refritos	7 oz	326	18	44	525	13	10.0	22.0	5	27%
Mexican rice	4 oz	159	3	30	530	1	2.0	0.0	1	12%
TACO										
chicken, soft	7 oz	387	21	41	933	7	16.0	48.0	6	37%
crisp	4 oz	295	22	16	609	5	17.0	48.0	7	50%
flour, soft, rolled	7 oz	512	33	46	1111	12	23.0	63.0	10	40%
meat	2.5 oz	208	22	7	576	5	11.0	38.0	4	46%
meat, natural, 'Super'	11.25 oz	627	41	60	915	14	27.0	82.0	13	38%
shredded beef, soft, 'Super'	8 oz	368	12	38	556	7	11.0	22.0	6	33%
soft, 'Value'	5.25 oz	316	24	23	599	5	15.0	48.0	7	42%
TACO SHELL, 6-inch	1.25 oz	110	2	14	48	2	6.0	0.0	1	46%
TOMATO	0.5 oz	3	0	1	1	0	0.0	0.0	0	0%
TORTILLA										
flour, 10-inch	2.75 oz	213	6	31	393	6	4.0	0.0	1	20%
flour, 8-inch	1.25 oz	107	5	16	33	2	3.0	0.0	1	24%
flour, 7-inch	1.75 oz	88	4	16	42	1	1.0	0.0	0	10%
flour, fried, 10-inch	2.75 oz	318	6	37	315	2	16.0	0.0	4	46%
flour, fried, 8-inch	1.3 oz	205	4	24	203	1	11.0	0.0	2	47%
wheat, 11-inch	3.5 oz	175	8	33	84	2	3.0	0.0	1	14%
WENDY'S										
BACON	1 slice	20	2	0	65	0	1.5	5.0	0	63%
BEVERAGE										
coffee	6 fl oz	0	0	1	0	0	0.0	0.0	0	0%
coffee, decaffeinated	6 fl oz	0	0	1	0	0	0.0	0.0	0	0%
cola, diet, small	8 fl oz	0	0	0	20	0	0.0	0.0	0	0%
cola, regular, small	8 fl oz	90	0	24	10	0	0.0	0.0	0	0%

Food Name	Serv. Size	Total Cal.	Prot. gms	Carbs gms	Sod. mgs	Fiber gms	Fat gms	Chol. mgs	Sat.Fat gms	%Fat Cal.
'Frosty' large	20 oz	540	14	91	320	0	14.0	60.0	9	23%
'Frosty' medium	16 oz	440	11	73	260	0	11.0	50.0	7	23%
'Frosty' small	12 oz	330	8	56	200	0	8.0	35.0	5	22%
hot chocolate	6 fl oz	80	1	15	135	0	3.0	0.0	0	30%
lemonade, small	8 fl oz	90	0	24	5	0	0.0	0.0	0	0%
lemon-lime soft drink	8 fl oz	90	0	24	25	0	0.0	0.0	0	0%
milk, 2%	8 fl oz	110	8	11	115	0	4.0	15.0	3	32%
tea, hot or iced	6 fl oz	0	0	0	0	0	0.0	0.0	0	0%
BREAD, pita, 'Classic Greek'	1 pita	440	15	50	1050	4	20.0	35.0	8	41%
BREADSTICK, soft	1 stick	130	4	23	250	1	3.0	5.0	1	20%
BUN										
Kaiser	1 bun	190	6	36	340	2	3.0	0.0	1	14%
sandwich	1 bun	160	5	29	280	2	2.5	0.0	1	14%
CHEESE										
American	1 slice	70	3	1	320	0	5.0	15.0	4	74%
American, junior	1 slice	45	2	0	220	0	3.5	10.0	3	80%
Cheddar, shredded	2 tbsp	70	4	1	110	0	6.0	15.0	4	73%
imitation, shredded, salad bar item	2 tbsp	50	3	1	260	0	4.0	0.0	1	69%
CHEESEBURGER										
bacon, junior	1 burger	380	20	34	850	2	19.0	60.0	7	44%
deluxe, junior	1 burger	360	18	36	890	3	17.0	50.0	6	41%
junior	1 burger	320	17	34	830	2	13.0	45.0	6	36%
kid's meal	1 burger	320	17	33	830	2	13.0	45.0	6	37%
CHICKEN										
fillet, breaded	1 piece	230	22	10	490	0	12.0	55.0	3	46%
fillet, grilled	1 fillet	110	22	0	450	0	3.0	60.0	1	23%
fillet, spicy	1 piece	210	22	10	920	0	9.0	60.0	2	39%
nuggets, fried	5 pieces	210	14	7	460	0	14.0	45.0	3	60%
nuggets, fried	4 pieces	170	11	5	370	0	11.0	35.0	3	61%
CHILI										
large	12 oz	310	23	32	1190	7	10.0	45.0	4	29%
small	8 oz	210	15	21	800	5	7.0	30.0	3	30%
CONDIMENTS. See also Salad Dressing.										
bacon bits, salad bar item	2 tbsp	45	6	0	550	0	2.5	10.0	1	48%
barbecue sauce	1 packet	45	1	10	160	0	0.0	0.0	0	0%
buffalo wing sauce, spicy	1 packet	25	0	4	210	0	1.0	0.0	0	36%
catsup	1 tsp	10	0	2	75	0	0.0	0.0	0	0%
croutons, salad bar item	2 tbsp	14	1	4	65	0	1.0	0.0	0	31%
honey mustard sauce	1 packet	130	0	6	220	0	12.0	10.0	2	82%
honey mustard, lower calorie	1 tsp	25	0	2	45	0	1.5	0.0	0	63%
lettuce	1 leaf	0	0	0	0	0	0.0	0.0	0	0%
lettuce, iceberg/Romaine, salad bar item	1 cup	10	0	2	5	1	0.0	0.0	0	0%
margarine, whipped	1 packet	60	0	0	115	0	7.0	0.0	2	100%
mayonnaise	1 tsp	30	0	1	60	0	3.0	5.0	0	87%
mustard	1 tsp	0	0	0	50	0	0.0	0.0	0	0%
onion, red, sliced, salad bar item	3 rings	0	0	1	0	0	0.0	0.0	0	0%
onion, sliced	4 rings	5	0	1	0	0	0.0	0.0	0	0%
Parmesan blend, grated, salad bar item	2 tbsp	70	4	5	290	0	4.0	10.0	2	50%
pepperoni, sliced, salad bar item	6 slices	30	1	0	70	0	3.0	5.0	1	87%

Food Name	Serv. Size	Total Cal.	Prot. gms	Carbs gms	Sod. mgs	Fiber gms	Fat gms	Chol. mgs	Sat.Fat gms	%Fat Cal.
pickle	4 slices	0	0	0	140	0	0.0	0.0	0	0%
salad oil	1 tbsp	120	0	0	0	0	14.0	0.0	2	100%
sour cream	1 packet	60	1	1	15	0	6.0	10.0	4	87%
sunflower seeds and raisins, salad bar item	2 tbsp	80	0	5	0	1	5.0	0.0	1	69%
sweet and sour sauce	1 packet	50	0	12	120	0	0.0	0.0	0	0%
tomato, sliced	1 slice	5	0	1	0	0	0.0	0.0	0	0%
tomato, wedges, salad bar item	1 piece	5	0	1	0	0	0.0	0.0	0	0%
turkey ham, diced, salad bar item	2 tbsp	50	3	0	280	0	4.0	25.0	1	75%
COOKIE, chocolate chip	1 cookie	270	3	36	120	1	13.0	30.0	6	43%
CRACKERS, saltine	2 crackers	25	1	4	80	0	0.5	0.0	0	18%
HAMBURGER										
'Big Bacon Classic'	1 burger	580	34	46	1460	3	30.0	100.0	12	46%
junior	1 burger	270	15	34	610	2	10.0	30.0	4	31%
kid's meal	1 burger	270	15	33	610	2	10.0	30.0	4	32%
single, plain	1 burger	360	24	31	580	2	16.0	65.0	6	40%
w/everything	1 burger	420	25	37	920	3	20.0	70.0	7	42%
HAMBURGER PATTY										
regular	2 oz	100	9	0	150	0	7.0	30.0	3	64%
quarter-pound	0.25 lb	200	19	0	290	0	14.0	65.0	6	62%
SALAD										
Caesar, side	1 salad	100	8	8	620	1	4.0	10.0	2	36%
chicken Caesar	1 salad	260	26	17	1170	2	9.0	60.0	3	32%
chicken, grilled	1 salad	200	25	9	720	3	8.0	50.0	2	35%
garden, deluxe	1 salad	110	7	9	350	3	6.0	0.0	1	46%
side	1 salad	60	4	5	180	2	3.0	0.0	0	43%
taco	1 salad	380	26	28	1040	7	19.0	65.0	10	44%
SALAD DRESSING										
blue cheese	2 tbsp	180	1	0	180	0	19.0	15.0	4	98%
Caesar vinaigrette, pita dressing	1 tbsp	70	0	1	170	0	7.0	0.0	1	94%
French	2 tbsp	120	0	6	330	0	10.0	0.0	2	79%
French, nonfat	2 tbsp	35	0	8	150	0	0.0	0.0	0	0%
garden ranch, pita dressing	1 tbsp	50	0	1	125	0	4.5	10.0	1	91%
Italian Caesar	2 tbsp	150	1	1	240	0	16.0	20.0	3	95%
Italian, reduced fat	2 tbsp	40	0	2	340	0	3.0	0.0	0	77%
ranch, 'Hidden Valley'	2 tbsp	100	1	1	220	0	10.0	10.0	2	92%
ranch, reduced fat, 'Hidden Valley'	2 tbsp	60	1	2	240	0	5.0	10.0	1	79%
Thousand Island	2 tbsp	90	0	2	125	0	8.0	10.0	2	90%
wine vinegar	1 tbsp	0	0	0	0	0	0.0	0.0	0	0%
SANDWICH										
chicken, breaded	1 sandwich	440	28	44	840	2	18.0	60.0	4	36%
chicken, grilled	1 sandwich	310	27	35	790	2	8.0	65.0	2	23%
chicken, spicy	1 sandwich	410	28	43	1280	2	15.0	65.0	3	32%
chicken Caesar pita	1 pita	490	34	48	1320	4	18.0	65.0	5	33%
chicken club	1 sandwich	470	31	44	970	2	20.0	70.0	4	38%
'Garden Ranch Chicken Pita'	1 pita	480	30	51	1180	5	18.0	70.0	4	33%
'Garden Veggie Pita'	1 pita	400	11	52	760	5	17.0	20.0	4	38%
SIDE DISH										
applesauce, salad bar item	2 tbsp	30	0	7	0	0	0.0	0.0	0	0%
baked potato, plain	10 oz	310	7	71	25	7	0.0	0.0	0	0%

Food Name	Serv. Size	Total Cal.	Prot. gms	Carbs gms	Sod. mgs	Fiber gms	Fat gms	Chol. mgs	Sat.Fat gms	%Fat Cal.
baked potato, w/bacon and cheese	1 serving	530	17	78	1390	7	18.0	20.0	4	30%
baked potato, w/broccoli and cheese ...	1 serving	470	9	80	470	9	14.0	5.0	3	26%
baked potato, w/cheese	1 serving	570	14	78	640	7	23.0	30.0	8	36%
baked potato, w/chili and cheese	1 serving	630	20	83	770	9	24.0	40.0	9	34%
baked potato, w/sour cream and chives	1 serving	380	8	74	40	8	6.0	15.0	4	14%
cantaloupe, sliced, salad bar item	1 piece	15	0	4	0	0	0.0	0.0	0	0%
chicken salad, salad bar item	2 tbsp	70	4	2	135	0	5.0	0.0	1	65%
cottage cheese, salad bar item	2 tbsp	30	4	1	125	0	1.5	5.0	1	40%
cucumbers, salad bar item	2 slices	0	0	0	0	0	0.0	0.0	0	0%
egg, hard cooked, salad bar item	2 tbsp	40	3	0	30	0	3.0	110.0	1	69%
french fries, 'Biggie'	5.6 oz	470	6	61	150	6	23.0	0.0	4	44%
french fries, 'Great Biggie'	6.7 oz	570	8	73	180	7	27.0	0.0	4	43%
french fries, small	3.2 oz	270	4	35	85	3	13.0	0.0	2	43%
green peas, salad bar item	2 tbsp	15	1	3	25	1	0.0	0.0	0	0%
green peppers, salad bar item	2 pieces	0	0	1	0	0	0.0	0.0	0	0%
orange, sliced, salad bar item	2 slices	15	0	4	0	1	0.0	0.0	0	0%
pasta salad, salad bar item	2 tbsp	35	1	4	180	1	1.5	0.0	0	40%
peaches, sliced, salad bar item	1 piece	15	0	4	0	0	0.0	0.0	0	0%
potato salad, salad bar item	2 tbsp	80	0	5	180	0	7.0	5.0	3	76%
watermelon, wedges, salad bar item	1 piece	20	0	4	0	0	0.0	0.0	0	0%
TACO CHIPS	15 chips	210	3	24	180	2	11.0	0.0	2	48%

WHATABURGER

Food Name	Serv. Size	Total Cal.	Prot. gms	Carbs gms	Sod. mgs	Fiber gms	Fat gms	Chol. mgs	Sat.Fat gms	%Fat Cal.
BACON	1 slice	38	2	0	106	na	3.3	6.0	na	79%
BEVERAGE										
'Cherry Coke' medium	1 serving	227	0	60	11	na	0.0	0.0	na	0%
chocolate shake, junior	1 serving	364	9	61	172	na	9.3	36.0	na	23%
'Coca-Cola Classic' medium	1 serving	211	0	56	19	na	0.0	0.0	na	0%
coffee, small	1 serving	5	0	1	5	na	0.0	0.0	na	0%
'Diet Coke' medium	1 serving	2	0	1	26	na	0.0	0.0	na	0%
'Dr Pepper' medium	1 serving	207	0	52	51	na	0.0	0.0	na	0%
iced tea, 'Lipton' medium	1 serving	5	0	2	15	na	0.0	0.0	na	0%
orange juice, 'Tropicana'	10 fl oz	140	2	33	0	na	0.0	0.0	na	0%
milk, 2%	1 serving	113	8	11	113	na	4.3	18.0	na	34%
'Sprite' medium	1 serving	211	0	48	45	na	0.0	0.0	na	0%
strawberry shake, junior	1 serving	352	9	60	168	na	8.9	35.0	na	23%
root beer, medium	1 serving	237	0	63	25	na	0.0	0.0	na	0%
vanilla shake, junior	1 serving	325	9	51	172	na	9.5	37.0	na	26%
BISCUIT, plain	1 serving	280	5	37	509	na	13.4	3.0	na	42%
BREAKFAST										
bacon biscuit	1 sandwich	359	10	37	730	na	20.2	15.0	na	50%
bacon, egg, and cheese biscuit	1 sandwich	511	18	38	1010	na	32.9	213.0	na	57%
'Breakfast on a Bun' w/bacon biscuit	1 sandwich	365	18	29	815	na	19.4	210.0	na	48%
Breakfast on a Bun' w/sausage biscuit	1 sandwich	455	20	30	886	na	28.1	232.0	na	56%
cinnamon roll	1 serving	320	4	39	190	na	16.0	10.0	na	46%
egg and cheese biscuit	1 sandwich	434	14	38	797	na	26.3	202.0	na	54%
egg omelet sandwich	1 sandwich	288	13	29	602	na	12.8	198.0	na	40%

Food Name	Serv. Size	Total Cal.	Prot. gms	Carbs gms	Sod. mgs	Fiber gms	Fat gms	Chol. mgs	Sat.Fat gms	%Fat Cal.
pancake	3 pancakes	259	11	40	842	na	5.8	0.0	na	21%
pancake, 3 pancakes w/1 sausage patty	1 serving	426	18	40	1127	na	21.1	34.0	na	45%
pancake, 3 pancakes w/2 slices bacon	1 serving	335	15	40	1074	na	12.4	12.0	na	34%
platter, w/bacon, scrambled eggs, biscuit, hash browns	1 serving	695	22	54	1162	na	44.0	389.0	na	57%
platter, w/sausage, scrambled eggs, biscuit, hash browns	1 serving	785	25	54	1234	na	52.7	412.0	na	60%
sausage and gravy biscuit	1 sandwich	479	9	48	1253	na	27.4	20.0	na	52%
sausage biscuit	1 sandwich	446	12	37	794	na	28.7	37.0	na	57%
sausage, egg, and cheese biscuit	1 sandwich	601	21	38	1081	na	41.6	236.0	na	62%
toast, Texas	1 slice	147	4	22	250	na	4.5	0.0	na	28%
CHEESE, large slice	1 slice	89	5	0	338	na	7.4	22.0	na	75%
CHICKEN STRIPS	2 strips	300	16	15	630	na	20.0	35.0	na	59%
COOKIE										
chocolate chunk	1 serving	247	4	28	75	na	16.0	36.0	na	53%
white chocolate macadamia nut	1 serving	269	3	31	80	na	16.0	34.0	na	51%
FAJITA										
beef	1 serving	326	22	34	670	na	11.9	28.0	na	33%
chicken, grilled	1 serving	272	18	35	691	na	6.7	33.0	na	22%
GRAVY, peppered	3 oz	75	0	8	375	na	4.5	0.0	na	57%
HAMBURGER										
'Justaburger'	1 burger	298	15	30	598	na	13.0	42.0	na	39%
'Whataburger'	1 burger	598	30	61	1096	na	26.0	84.0	na	39%
'Whataburger' double meat	1 burger	823	49	62	1298	na	42.4	168.0	na	46%
'Whataburger Jr.'	1 burger	322	16	35	603	na	13.3	42.0	na	37%
'Whataburger' on small bun, w/o oil	1 burger	407	25	34	839	na	18.8	84.0	na	42%
MUFFIN, blueberry	1 serving	239	6	36	538	na	7.9	0.0	na	30%
SALAD										
garden	1 salad	56	3	11	32	na	0.6	0.0	na	9%
chicken, grilled	1 salad	150	23	14	434	na	1.2	49.0	na	7%
SANDWICH										
chicken, grilled	1 sandwich	442	34	48	1103	na	14.2	66.0	na	28%
chicken, grilled, on small white bun, w/mustard, w/o oil, dressing	1 sandwich	300	33	35	994	na	3.2	66.0	na	10%
chicken, grilled, w/o dressing	1 sandwich	385	34	46	989	na	8.5	66.0	na	19%
chicken, grilled, w/o dressing, oil	1 sandwich	358	34	46	989	na	5.5	66.0	na	13%
fish, 'Whatacatch'	1 sandwich	467	18	43	636	na	25.0	33.0	na	48%
SIDE DISH										
french fries, junior	1 serving	221	4	25	139	na	12.1	0.0	na	49%
french fries, large	1 serving	442	7	49	227	na	24.2	0.0	na	49%
french fries, regular	1 serving	332	5	37	208	na	18.1	0.0	na	49%
onion rings, large	1 serving	498	8	51	893	na	28.7	0.0	na	52%
onion rings, regular	1 serving	329	5	34	596	na	19.1	0.0	na	52%
TAQUITO										
bacon and egg	1 serving	335	15	32	761	na	16.1	286.0	na	44%
potato and egg	1 serving	446	14	48	883	na	21.8	281.0	na	44%
sausage and egg	1 serving	443	20	32	790	na	25.9	315.0	na	53%

Food Name	Serv. Size	Total Cal.	Prot. gms	Carbs gms	Sod. mgs	Fiber gms	Fat gms	Chol. mgs	Sat.Fat gms	%Fat Cal.
TURNOVER, apple, fried	1 serving	215	2	27	241	na	10.8	0.0	na	45%

WHITE CASTLE
BEVERAGE

Food Name	Serv. Size	Total Cal.	Prot. gms	Carbs gms	Sod. mgs	Fiber gms	Fat gms	Chol. mgs	Sat.Fat gms	%Fat Cal.
chocolate shake	14 fl oz	220	8	32	140	0	7.0	25.0	1	28%
'Coca-Cola Classic'	14 fl oz	120	0	32	12	0	0.0	0.0	0	0%
coffee, black, small	1 serving	6	0	1	5	0	0.0	0.0	0	0%
'Diet Coke'	14 fl oz	1	0	0	13	0	0.0	0.0	0	0%
tea, iced	14 fl oz	45	0	12	15	0	0.0	0.0	0	0%
vanilla shake	14 fl oz	230	8	35	150	0	7.0	25.0	1	27%

BREAKFAST, egg, sausage, cheese

Food Name	Serv. Size	Total Cal.	Prot. gms	Carbs gms	Sod. mgs	Fiber gms	Fat gms	Chol. mgs	Sat.Fat gms	%Fat Cal.
on bun	1 sandwich	340	14	17	900	0	25.0	130.0	10	64%

CHEESEBURGER

Food Name	Serv. Size	Total Cal.	Prot. gms	Carbs gms	Sod. mgs	Fiber gms	Fat gms	Chol. mgs	Sat.Fat gms	%Fat Cal.
double patty	1 sandwich	285	14	16	430	5	18.0	30.0	8	57%
regular	1 sandwich	160	7	11	250	2	9.0	15.0	4	53%
w/bacon	1 sandwich	200	10	12	400	3	13.0	25.0	6	57%
CHICKEN RINGS	6 rings	310	16	14	620	0	21.0	70.0	4	61%
CHILI	12 oz	375	30	45	1635	0	15.0	0.0	0	31%

HAMBURGER

Food Name	Serv. Size	Total Cal.	Prot. gms	Carbs gms	Sod. mgs	Fiber gms	Fat gms	Chol. mgs	Sat.Fat gms	%Fat Cal.
double	1 burger	235	11	16	200	4	14.0	20.0	6	54%
regular	1 burger	135	6	11	135	2	7.0	10.0	3	48%

SANDWICH

Food Name	Serv. Size	Total Cal.	Prot. gms	Carbs gms	Sod. mgs	Fiber gms	Fat gms	Chol. mgs	Sat.Fat gms	%Fat Cal.
chicken	1 sandwich	190	8	21	360	0	8.0	20.0	2	38%
fish	1 sandwich	160	8	18*	220	0	6.0	15.0	1	34%

SIDE DISH

Food Name	Serv. Size	Total Cal.	Prot. gms	Carbs gms	Sod. mgs	Fiber gms	Fat gms	Chol. mgs	Sat.Fat gms	%Fat Cal.
cheese sticks	3 sticks	290	15	19	730	0	17.0	0.0	5	53%
french fries, small	1 serving	115	0	15	15	2	6.0	0.0	1	47%
onion rings	8 rings	540	8	69	1300	0	26.0	0.0	0	43%

Nutrition and Fitness Software for Your Windows PC

Looking to save time and effort managing your nutrition and exercise? If you have a Windows computer (Win 95 and up), you're in luck.

NutriBase nutrition and fitness software provides you with a research-quality nutrient database that gives you instant access to more than 100 nutrients. In fact, the data used in the NutriBase series of books is a subset of the data contained in the NutriBase software.

The software will allow you to view, rank, query, and perform food name searches on the nutrient data. You can track your dietary intake; create and analyze recipes; record and track your exercise; count calories, carbs, protein, or any other nutrient; add new food items, create meals; generate meal plans; graph results; generate reports; and monitor your progress on a daily basis.

For complete product information, free downloads, and links to our competitors, visit us at:

NutriBase EZ Edition (easy-to-use edition)   imchubby.com

NutriBase Personal Plus Edition (robust personal edition)   dietsoftware.com

NutriBase Clinical Edition (professional nutrition software)   nutribase.com

Cybersoft, Inc. (800) 959-4849